WOMEN MAKING HISTORY

WOMEN AND HEALTH

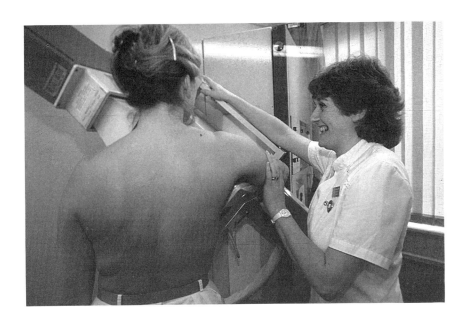

PAT HODGSON

B. T. Batsford Ltd   London

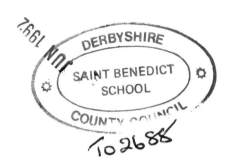

Frontispiece
A woman is screened for cancer.

Cover illustrations
Colour: a woman enjoys an aerobic workout;
background: a hospital waiting room around 1910.

Typeset by Tek-Art Ltd, West Wickham, Kent
and printed in Great Britain
by The Bath Press, Bath
for the publishers
B. T. Batsford Ltd
4 Fitzhardinge Street
London W1H 0AH

ISBN 0 7134 6295 7

Acknowledgements

The Author and Publishers would like to thank the
following for permission to reproduce illustrations:
Bibliothèque Nationale, Paris for page 4; BMA News
Review for page 59b; Brook Advisory Centre for page
16; City Syndication Ltd for page 50; Sally and
Richard Greenhill for page 29, 36b, 51, 54;
Greenpeace/Morgan for page 28; Pat Hodgson
Library for pages 6, 9, 10, 11, 14, 20, 22b, 24, 31, 36a,
41, 47, 53, 59a; Hulton Picture Company for pages 13,
22a, 23, 27, 34, 39, 43, 58; Diana Lamplugh for pages
37, 45; Monitor Press Features for page 56; Maggie
Murray/Format Photographers for page 48; Susie
Orbach for page 19; Posy Simmonds for page 17; The
Women's National Cancer Control Campaign for
page 60.

Contents

Introduction

The reason for having a book about Women and Health, rather than discussing pioneers of both genders, is that family health was initially thought to be a mother's responsibility. Women in the past were expected to be a combination of doctor, nurse and pharmacist in the home. They were therefore uniquely qualified to become professionals when opportunities to work in health-related professions became available to them from the late nineteenth century. By this time the public figures associated with health – doctors, surgeons, nutritionists and public health legislators – were all men. Within the home women cared for the sick, cooked food, cleaned the house, looked after children and concocted folk remedies for ailments. However, women had always had their place in the

1 Nuns helped to care for the sick in the Middle Ages.

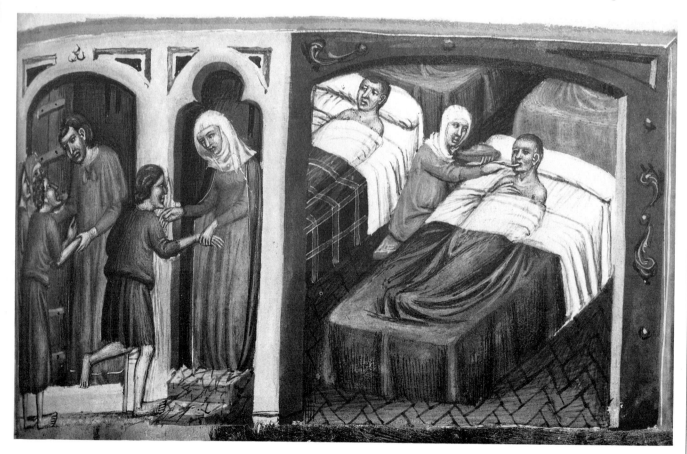

community as midwives, healers, pharmacists and even doctors at a non-professional level. In the sixteenth and seventeenth centuries some of these women were suspected of witchcraft – a Scottish midwife was executed in 1591 for supposedly using magical means to ease pain during labour.

The development of male and female roles in medicine was the result of ingrained social attitudes towards women. In the past women had few rights in law and often had the status of chief servant at home. Women were excluded from university education until the late nineteenth century, effectively preventing them from training as doctors.

> The doctor-nurse-patient relationship in and out of hospital is largely based on that which usually obtains at ward level. That relationship mirrors the stereotype of the bourgeois family where father dominates and performs the role of decision-taker and protector whilst mother's role is passive, consisting of servicing activities and carrying out the wishes of the father. (*Woman & Medicine*)

Although women often acted as unpaid doctors, nurses and herbalists in the past, they themselves had little treatment if they were ill. Women's gynaecological problems and other 'female complaints', which were often caused by childbirth or malnutrition, generally went untreated up to the time of the National Health Service. There were few women doctors and many women were too frightened or shy to consult men. Even pregnancy had to be concealed under voluminous clothes in Victorian Britain. Gynaecology did not become a recognized speciality until 1929. Alma Rosser remembered her family's attitude to doctors in the 1920s:

> Anything from the waist down was absolutely taboo. And I suppose my grandparents would be afraid to go to the doctor. . . there was a certain amount of embarrassment and shame about women's illnesses. (Quoted in *Out of the Doll's House*)

Lack of efficient methods of birth control led to large families, and many babies died at birth because of insanitary conditions. Mothers died of puerperal fever before the discovery of antibiotics at the end of the Second World War. Rich women could afford to pay for professional attention before the National Health Service but the poor were at the mercy of 'quack' remedies. Abortionists and the makers of patent medicines advertised in newspapers and many strange potions gained the reputation for terminating a

pregnancy. Sanatogen Tonic Wine was advertised widely as a cure for most minor ailments – even teetotallers used to drink it.

Kathleen Dayus remembers some of her mother's cures for common illnesses, just before the First World War:

> Headaches, we had vinegar and brown paper; for whooping cough we had camphorated oil rubbed on our chests or goose fat. For mumps we had stockings round our throats and measles we had tea stewed in the teapot by the fire . . . (Quoted in *Out of the Doll's House*)

Little attention was paid to the poor physical condition of British people until recruits were needed for the Boer War and few men reached the minimum standard of health. A report was published in 1904 after the Boer War in which the authorities blamed women for not giving their babies the correct food, rather than placing the blame on the real causes – bad housing, poverty, and the economic position of women, who were dependent on the 'housekeeping' money given to them by their husbands. School meals for poor children commenced in 1906 and the following year regular medical inspections were started. In future, schools were to teach infant care as well as domestic science. The National Health Insurance Act of 1911, which provided the first state health care in Britain, was for workers earning under £160 a year. Treatment could be obtained free of charge from a 'panel' doctor, but generally only the men qualified – their wives and children still had to pay or go without.

Attention was drawn to the poor state of women's health by another war. Women, who took the place of men in the munitions factories during the First World War, were often too ill to work properly. Factory welfare supervisors were appointed by the government, and at the end of the war the Maternal and Child Welfare Act set up free clinics for pregnant women and infants. Poverty and bad housing, however, continued, and it took another war for the National Health Service to be established.

The National Health Service Act, which became law in 1948, raised the standard of women's health generally. At last able to consult a doctor freely, women could obtain help for their chronic and often serious conditions. Regular innoculations resulted in fewer child deaths from infectious diseases. Free school meals, milk and orange juice meant that all children were better nourished. The post-Second

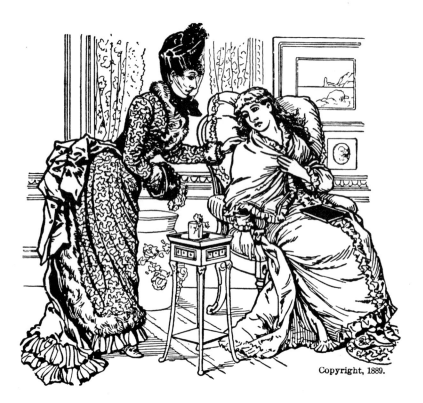

Copyright, 1889.

2 An 1889 advertisement for Dr Pierce's Favourite Prescription: 'The world-famed remedy for all those chronic weaknesses and distressing derangements so common to women'.

World War was also easier for women in other ways. Various labour-saving devices and kitchen appliances gradually came on to the market, and many women now had jobs which helped to pay for them. New houses were built with central heating and bathrooms.

The emancipation of women brought with it other benefits to their health. As women went out to work, so the social conventions changed and, with them, Victorian attitudes to dress, exercise and sex. Women's clothes became lighter and more comfortable and regular exercise became a more common part of their lives. Advice on contraception became freely obtainable from doctors or Well-Woman clinics. Emancipa-

tion also had its disadvantages. Although stress is not suffered only by people in top management jobs, or indeed any job at all, professional women are beginning to develop the type of stress-related illnesses once more often associated with men. We are today living in the most health-conscious age, and yet there are new problems like environmental pollution and even new diseases to combat.

CHAPTER 1

The Pioneers

Florence Nightingale (1820–1910)

Florence Nightingale was an attractive, intelligent girl who came from a privileged background. Her parents were appalled when she decided at the age of 25 to become a nurse at Kaiserswerth – a religious community in Germany. She had come to her decision because she felt called by God to help the sick and believed that nursing was the practical way of carrying this out.

Although professional nurses existed in the mid-nineteenth century, there was no recognized training, and middle-class parents never thought the occupation suitable for their daughters. Most of the work was purely domestic; caring for strangers in bed was immodest in Victorian eyes, and nurses had an unfortunate reputation for drunkenness and immorality. Although these criticisms naturally did not apply to nursing orders of nuns like those at Kaiserswerth, Florence Nightingale's parents had other plans for their daughter. In later life she said, 'It was as if I wanted to be a kitchen maid'.

Florence Nightingale was very determined. She persisted in her plan, studied at Kaiserswerth, and was working as superintendent of a home for sick gentlewomen when the Crimean War broke out in 1854. When she read in *The Times* how the wounded were suffering, she persuaded an old friend, Sidney Herbert, by this time War Secretary, to arrange for her to go to the Crimea with a small party of 40 experienced nurses, personally selected by her from hospitals and convents. When she arrived, she was horrified by the conditions she found there.

It is with feelings of surprise and anger that the public will learn that no sufficient preparations have been made for the

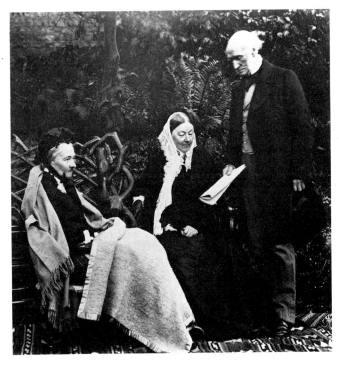

3 *Florence Nightingale (centre) at Claydon with her sister Parthenope and Sir Harry Verney in about 1890.*

proper care of the wounded. Not only are there not sufficient surgeons . . . not only are there no dressers and nurses . . . but what will be said when it is known that there is not even linen to make bandages for the wounded. (William Howard Russell, writing in the *Times*, 12 October 1854.)

Ms Nightingale is remembered today for her work as a nurse in the Crimean War. In fact, her influence was much wider, extending to cover all aspects of soldiers' welfare – diet, cleanliness, hospital buildings, allocation of supplies, disposal of sewage and personal problems. In the muddle of war created by an inept War Office, she had a genius for cutting through red tape and achieving results. She made some enemies among the generals and Royal Army Medical Corps surgeons, but the soldiers loved her. Queen Victoria followed her progress with great interest, and she became the heroine of the British people.

> She is a 'ministering angel' without any exaggeration in these hospitals, and as her slender form glides quietly along each corridor, every poor fellow's face softens with gratitude at the sight of her. When all the medical officers have retired for the night and silence and darkness have settled down upon those miles of prostrate sick, she may be observed alone, with a little lamp in her hand, making her solitary rounds. (Mr Macdonald, commissioner of *The Times* Fund)

Her experiences in the Crimean War led Ms Nightingale to make two vows which she tried to fulfil throughout the rest of her life. One was to make nursing into a profession with recognized training and the other was to improve the general and medical welfare of peacetime soldiers. Her investigative mind tackled every kind of problem and she got through a formidable amount of work. Although receiving a little secretarial help from friends, she wrote most of her books, reports and letters longhand. Her private life was non-existent, her health suffered, and she soon found it better to remain at home – sometimes in bed – to write her reports and receive callers.

Florence's parents were not reconciled to her career. Although proud of her during the war, her mother and sister thought she would return home when peace came, perhaps marry, and if not, stay to look after her family. Although by this time consulted by Cabinet Ministers as the recognized authority on nursing and army matters, Ms Nightingale was constantly torn between the demands of her family and work. She did not become free of this moral dilemma until her mother died in 1880. With such a background, her achievements are even more remarkable.

Florence Nightingale considered her first priority after the war to be to improve conditions for peacetime soldiers, who had needlessly suffered so much during the war.

> I stand at the altar of the murdered men and, while I live, I fight their cause. (Florence Nightingale, 1856)

Her army reforms led to improved health for home and foreign-based soldiers, and she also took part in the detailed planning of military hospitals, pioneering the use of statistics in her reports. She was particularly concerned with conditions in India and confessed in later life that India remained 'the constant object of my thoughts'.

Of equal importance was Florence Nightingale's desire to make nursing into a respected profession for educated women. In 1860 the Nightingale School for training nurses opened at St Thomas's Hospital, based on Ms Nightingale's recommendations. Her advice on nursing practice and ward design, contained in her books *Notes on Nursing* and *Notes on Hospitals*, remains relevant today. Her comments are crisp and to the point. She believed above all that nurses should be practical, sensible and imaginative and that they should not shirk unpleasant jobs:

> . . . Women who wait for the housemaid to do this or for the charwoman to do that when patients are suffering have not the *making* of a nurse in them. (*Notes on Nursing*, 1859)

Ms Nightingale also advised on midwifery and on community nursing, and collaborated with William Rathbone in the training of pioneer district nurses. She believed that non-surgical cases should be treated at home:

> Hospitals are but an intermediate stage of civilisation . . . the ultimate object is to nurse all sick at home. (*The Times*, 14 April 1876)

Florence Nightingale was 90 when she died in 1910. She continued into old age advising on nursing matters and maintained her relationship with the Nightingale School, addressing new probationers each year. In 1907 she was the first woman to be given the Order of Merit. Her character was an interesting blend of nineteenth-century and modern woman. She gave middle-class women in particular an alternative to family and marriage as their lifestyle. She made her name in a man's world during a period when women were expected to sit modestly at home, yet was much respected by her male colleagues. She had a wide circle of like-minded friends of both sexes, with whom she corresponded all her life – among them the writer Harriet Martineau (1802-1876), novelist George Eliot (1819-1880) and the educationist and supporter of women's suffrage Barbara Bodichon (1827-1891).

On the other hand, Florence Nightingale did not

believe that women should compete professionally with men and become doctors. She wanted them to succeed in their own sphere, which she believed to be nursing. She refused to accept that there was any discrimination against women and declined John Stuart Mill's invitation to become a member of the first Committee on Women's Suffrage, believing that the vote would not improve women's position in society. However, Florence Nightingale stands out as one of the great health pioneers because of the extraordinary scope of her work, her vision and her dedication to pursuing her goals, whatever the cost.

Questions

1 Why do you think Florence Nightingale was so determined to become a nurse at any cost? Why did her family disapprove of her choice of career?

2 Why do you think she believed that women should stick to their own sphere of nursing and not try to complete with men to become doctors?

3 What was Mr Macdonald's opinion of Florence Nightingale (see the quotation on page 8)? How appropriate an image of her do you think this is?

The Right to practise

Florence Nightingale was not the only intelligent woman to resent the way her life had been mapped out in advance by Victorian social conventions. Others suffered from similar problems, but had managed to carve out their own careers in health-connected fields in spite of opposition. Among them were Elizabeth Fry (1780-1845) the prison reformer, Josephine Butler (1828-1906), who fought for the rights of prostitutes, and Octavia Hill (1838-1912), who helped to improve housing conditions for the poor. Middle-class women were also accustomed to giving their unpaid help to poor families. Improved public health was the constant preoccupation of Victorian legislators, who were having to cope with the problems brought about by the Industrial Revolution – overcrowded, insanitary towns and inadequate homes for agricultural workers, which had changed little since medieval times.

Medicine had not always been solely a male preserve, in spite of Ms Nightingale's view that it was more suitable for men to be doctors and women nurses. In 1588 Tomazine Scarlet was fined £10 for prescribing medicines. In the seventeenth and eighteenth centuries there were female amateur healers, herbalists, 'leech women' and prescribers of patent medicines. A certain Mrs Philips had a

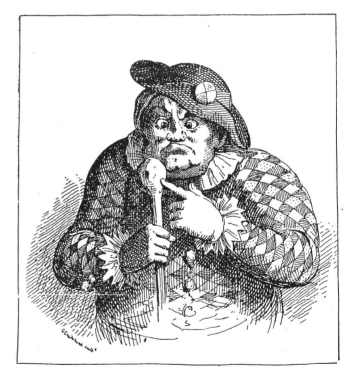

4 Mrs Sarah Mapp, the eighteenth-century bone setter (after a print by G. Cruikshank). Although an eccentric, Mrs Mapp was famous, and a contemporary wrote: 'Her bandages are extraordinary neat and her dexterity in reducing dislocations and setting fractured bones wonderful. The lame come to her daily and she gets a great deal of money'.

flourishing trade selling condoms made from dried sheep's gut in the seventeenth century, saying in her advertisement: 'Ambassadors, Foreigners, Gentlemen and Captains of Ships, may be supplied with any quantity' (quoted in *The Quacks of Old London*). Mrs Mapp was a highly successful bone-setter and unqualified orthopaedic surgeon in the eighteenth century. There were even one or two 'surgeonesses', who trained unofficially with the men. John Aubrey (1626-97) describes how Charles II was cured of a complaint by a 'she-surgeon'.

Most women preferred to consult someone of their own sex and the 'doctresses' generally specialized in female problems, childbirth and cosmetic remedies. Thomas Beddoes (1803-49) records that medical treatment was often performed by the doctor's wife – a practice he opposed. Dr 'James' Barry (1795-1865) was a woman who disguised herself as a man in order to qualify in medicine at Edinburgh in 1812, when she was only 17. She later joined the army, serving in South Africa, the Caribbean and the Crimean War. As a surgeon, she is credited with performing the first successful Caesarean section in South Africa in 1826 and had a formidable record at her various postings. When she died, her instructions that she should be buried without examination were ignored and her true sex was discovered as well as the fact that she had borne a child.

Elizabeth Blackwell (1821-1910) was the first woman in Britain to have her name on the medical register. She decided on the profession after a female friend had died of a 'uterine disorder', about which she had been too embarrased to consult her male doctor. After having failed to get in to a medical college in Britain, Elizabeth finally qualified at Geneva College in New York and gained hospital experience in Paris. She was forced to give up her ambition to train as a surgeon when an infection left her blind in one eye. She completed her training at St Bartholomew's Hospital, London, and then returned to America to practise.

The opposition to women doctors was not over. Although Elizabeth Blackwell was registered with the General Council of Medical Education and Registration in 1858, a new regulation was passed in 1860 stating that only women with English medical degrees could now register. As English universities still did not accept women undergraduates, this was an impossibility, and Elizabeth Garrett was only able to practise in 1865 by obtaining the Licentiate of the Society of Apothecaries and a Parisian degree.

In 1869 Sophie Jex Blake and four other women were accepted by the Edinburgh Medical School, but were subject to such harrassment that a separate women's school was founded in London. It was not until 1876 that teaching hospitals at last accepted female medical students. When both London and Edinburgh were refusing to accept female medical students in the early 1870s, thinking about the career of Dr James Barry, Alfred Swaine Taylor remarked:

> With such a successful precedent before them the examining board of Edinburgh are hardly justified in excluding women from professional study and examination. (Quoted in the *British Medical Journal*, Hurwitz & Richardson, 4 February 1989)

There had been many eminent women in the various branches of the nursing profession by the end of the nineteenth century, and not all were Nightingale trained. Mary Seacole, a Jamaican who had practised in her native country as a 'doctress', travelled to the Crimea at her own expense to nurse the troops, after arriving in London too late to go with Florence

5 A drawing of Mary Seacole by the Crimean War artist and correspondent William Simpson.

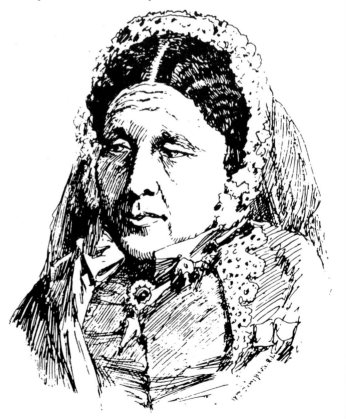

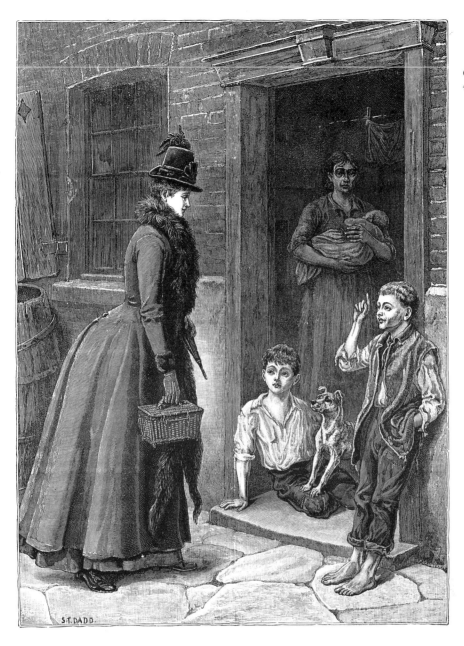

Nightingale's first party of nurses. She also provided stores and comforts, helping the wounded from the battlefield and giving them cups of tea while they waited for the boats to take them to hospital.

After the war, the soldiers remembered her with affection and a Benefit was held for her in 1857. When she died, *The Times* recognized that 'even in an enlightened century [she] stands out pre-eminent, and cannot be passed over'. In human terms her contribution was great, but unlike Florence Nightingale, her work had no lasting influence on the development of nursing or hospital administration.

She is often seen riding out to the front with baskets of medicines of her own preparation, and this is particularly the case after an engagement with the enemy. (*Morning Advertiser*, 19 July 1855)

Mrs Seacole published a book (*The Wonderful Adventures of Mrs Seacole in Many Lands*, 1857) and was awarded the Crimean medal.

Workhouse nursing had also been improved during the nineteenth century. Agnes Jones, one of Florence Nightingale's best nurses, became matron at the Liverpool Workhouse Infirmary in 1864 and did good work there before dying of typhus at a tragically young age in 1868.

What makes Workhouse nursing such an awful strain on all one's faculties is what made the War Hospital nursing so. It is not the hardship and the misery, but it is the struggle with all the authorities for justice . . . (Florence Nightingale to Madame Mohl, 1868)

Florence Nightingale had emphasized that improvements to the home environment were as important as hospital nursing, so that disease could be stopped at source. She supported the health visiting movement, which had originated in the Ladies Sanitary Reform Association, founded in Manchester and Salford in 1862. For the first time professional female health visitors advised on hygiene, diet and child care in the home. By the end of the nineteenth century in Britain there were qualified women doctors and professionally trained nurses, midwives and health visitors. In 1893 the first women factory inspectors were appointed, among them May Abraham and Mary Patterson, to look after the health of female workers.

Evidence

A But my chief occupation, and one with which I never allowed any business to interfere, was helping the doctors to transfer the sick and wounded from the mules and ambulances into the transports that had to carry them to the hospitals of Scutari and Buyukdere . . . With so many patients, the doctors must be glad of all the hands they could get. Indeed, so strong was the old impulse within me, that I waited for no permission, but seeing a poor artilleryman stretched upon a pallet, groaning heavily, I ran up to him at once, and eased the stiff dressings. Lightly my practised fingers ran over the familiar work, and well was I rewarded when the poor fellow's groans subsided into a restless uneasy mutter. God help him! He had been hit in the forehead and I think his sight was gone. I stooped down, and raised some tea to his baked lips . . . (Mary Seacole, *Wonderful Adventures of Mrs Seacole in Many Lands*)

B To every home sickness must come sooner or later, and it is to the women of the home that everyone turns when an accident or any other illness occurs. It is therefore the duty of every woman, nay, of every girl, to take some thought as to what she would be called upon to do should the emergency arise. Do not for a moment imagine that I would wish to cast any slur on that noble and devoted band of women, the trained hospital nurses, when I say that every girl should be taught to have some idea of nursing the sick . . . many slight illnesses, and many severe illnesses, could have been borne in greater comfort had the women of the household had the confidence of knowing what was the right thing to do . . . (*The Girls Own Paper*, 18 November 1905)

C We did twelve hours all night without a break and nothing to eat – I used to take cabbages from the garden. Sunday morning we got one sausage as a treat. We had to be in by ten and boys weren't allowed to say goodnight to you at the gate . . . If you had free time during the day you had to go to lectures. There was one doctor and he didn't speak to you until you were in the position of sister. (Mrs Shaw, who worked as a nurse in the early 1900s, quoted in Carol Adams, *Ordinary Lives*)

D We were all oddities to some extent. To be a medical student then you had to really want to do it. The Royal Free was the only hospital brave enough to take on women. We were the first women doctors any of the hospitals had had. They didn't know how to treat us . . . When the hospital got used to having women they found it was much better. The doctors could be friends with the sisters. Many women liked having women doctors too. (Dr Helena Wright, talking about her experiences prior to the First World War in Carol Adams, *Ordinary Lives*)

Questions

1 What experience had Mary Seacole had in dealing with the sick? Were the difficulties she had to contend with in the Crimea greater than those met with by Florence Nightingale?

2 Compare the status of women doctors and nurses, in C and D, at the beginning of the twentieth century. Were they treated in the same way? Why did hospitals have trouble getting used to women doctors?

3 What kind of picture do sources B, C and D present of women in medicine? How have things changed since then? Is anything still the same?

4 Why might people prefer to be treated by a woman today?

CHAPTER 2

Birth Control

Marie Stopes (1880–1956)

In my own marriage I paid such a terrible price for sex-ignorance that I feel knowledge gained at such a cost should be placed at the service of humanity. (Marie Stopes, *Married Love*, 1918)

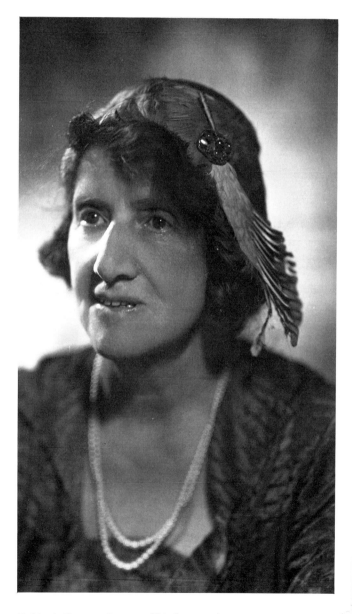

7 Marie Stopes, pioneer of birth control.

In common with many girls brought up before the First World War, Marie Stopes knew little about sex before she married Dr Reginald Gates at the age of 31. She was not happy and wondered why she had not become pregnant, when in fact the marriage had never been consummated. Her attempts to find an answer to her problems in books led to her first research into sexual matters. Seeing that the only chance to end her marriage was to plead non-consummation, she obtained an annulment, later marrying Humphrey Verdon Rowe. This second, happy marriage helped to formulate Marie Stopes's theories. Like a religious convert, she was eager to pass on to other women her knowledge about sexuality and to write a book of her own.

In other respects Marie Stopes had been well-educated. She obtained a degree in botany at University College and went on in 1903 to gain a doctorate at the Botanical Institute in Munich, where she was the only woman among 5000 men. Her first book, *Married Love*, published in 1918, put forward what was then a revolutionary idea – that sex within marriage was enjoyable for women as well as men.

Man, through prudery, through the custom of ignoring the woman's side of marriage and considering his own whim as marriage law, has largely lost the art of stirring a chaste partner to physical love. (Marie Stopes, *Married Love*)

Although the theme was scandalous at the time, 2000

copies of *Married Love* were sold in the first two weeks of publication. Many of Ms Stopes's ideas were not original, but the message that sex could be enjoyable and that society could be transformed if couples were sexually fulfilled was particularly important for women. Her second book, *Wise Parenthood*, published later in 1918, described methods of contraception and was addressed to married women only. In 1920 she suggested, in *Radiant Motherhood*, that women should have at least six weeks in bed after a baby was born.

Marie Stopes provided married women with a way of avoiding the health problems of a yearly pregnancy. Women could now limit the size of their families and for the first time feel in control of their bodies.

In 1921 Marie Stopes opened Britain's first birth control clinic at Holloway in London, where cervical caps were prescribed for women. There was opposition to her crusade from all sides on moral, religious, political and medical grounds.

> [She is] . . . responsible for providing instructions to girls of initially dubious virtue as to how to adopt the profession of more or less open prostitution. (Dr C.P. Blacker, 1924)

A female gynaecologist wrote:

> The mere discussion of contraceptive methods is lowering to the moral sense and to the innate reserve and purity of decently brought-up young people. (Dr Mary Scharlieb, quoted in *Marie Stopes: A Biography*)

Marie Stopes's aim was to make her clinic as respectable as possible to encourage women to attend. Running costs were paid by Ms Stopes and her husband, although there were a few donations of money. Patients were examined by a qualified midwife and a woman doctor visited the clinic once a week. Ms Stopes did not believe in abortion.

In the meantime, the Malthusian League had opened their own birth control clinic, the Walworth Women's Welfare Centre, which recommended the use of a diaphragm. Marie Stopes, who resented competition, resigned from the League and in 1921 founded the Society for Constructive Birth Control and Racial Progress.

In 1922 she took out a case for libel against Dr Halliday Sutherland, a Roman Catholic who had suggested in his book, *Birth Control: A Statement of Christian Doctrine against the New-Malthusians*, that the poor were being experimented on at birth control clinics. Although Ms Stopes finally lost the case when

it was taken to the House of Lords, the action created tremendous publicity and support for her cause.

Marie Stopes had a child in 1924 when she was 43, and in 1928 published *Enduring Passion*, advocating 'lifelong long and enduring monagamic devotion'. During the 1930s a number of provincial clinics were opened and Selfridges sponsored a caravan to tour the country giving advice on contraception. Many of the clinics continued until they were absorbed by local health authorities after the formation of the National Health Service in the late forties and early fifties.

Marie Stopes's contribution to women's health was immense. By bringing the subject of birth control into the open, she made a large contribution to making it respectable. And now, at last, there was someone impartial whom women could consult about their sex

8 A comic postcard about the inevitability of having large families in the Edwardian period.

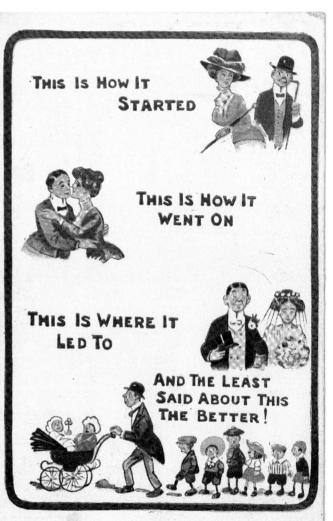

problems. She was a good publicist and she brought contraception to those who badly needed it. She always answered letters, many of which revealed the unhappy lives led by those with sexual or contraceptive problems. Although this kind of advice is freely available today, until Marie Stopes came along there was no one outside family and friends with whom women could discuss their problems.

Questions

1 Why were Marie Stopes's books, *Married Love* and *Wise Parenthood*, so popular?

2 What objections were raised to her birth control clinic?

3 Who benefited from Marie Stopes's pioneering action?

Contraception – The Woman's Choice

I should say that the majority of women are not very much troubled with sexual feeling of any kind. (William Acton, nineteenth century)

Sex was a forbidden topic in Victorian Britain and most girls were totally ignorant about the facts of life. Married women of all classes were constantly pregnant and many babies died at birth or in infancy. There was always the fear of having an illegitimate child which would result in social and economic ruin for a woman and even long engagements were often chaste. The only safe way to avoid an unwanted pregnancy was abstinence or abortion, which was illegal from 1861. Although some upper and middle-class families were trying to limit their families towards the end of the nineteenth century by using the condom, even in the 1920s many poor couples had little idea what to do or money to buy contraceptives. The Obscene Publications Act also prevented information about sex and birth control being freely available.

The two pioneers of birth control in the early twentieth century were Marie Stopes in Britain and Margaret Sanger (1879-1966) in America. Both were committed to providing contraception for the poor. The feminist Dora Russell also campaigned for birth control for working-class mothers and in 1923 was prosecuted for publishing explicit advice on the subject. When Mary Stocks and Charis Frankenburg opened a clinic in 1926 in Salford, there was strong opposition from the Catholics, who called them 'painted women of the worst kind'. But by persevering in their campaigning, these women began to change

attitudes to birth control. Women began to demand state provision of birth control for married women.

Between the wars many women were forced to have an abortion for social or economic reasons, often endangering their lives.

> There were various types of pills that were sold – pills to regulate you – and some were really poisonous. Some were just strong laxatives, but others would contain lead which, of course, is a disaster . . . They would buy these from shops – the rather doubtful shops which sold 'feminine pills'. (Dame Josephine Barnes, quoted in *Out of the Doll's House*)

One Salford woman remembers that during the 1920s Beecham's pills were recommended among her friends as an abortive.

> Beecham's used to be advertised as worth a guinea a box, the same price as a back street abortion in Salford. (Beatrice Sandys, quoted in *Out of the Doll's House*)

The National Birth Control Association was formed in 1931 to 'enable the poorer woman to obtain the advice now available for women rich enough to pay a specialist's fee'. The NCB provided special training for doctors and nurses, as none was given in medical schools. In 1939 the Association changed its name to the Family Planning Association, as the emphasis was now on family limitation for the sake of a woman's health.

Although moral attitudes became more relaxed as a result of the Second World War, when the National Health Service was formed in 1948 there was no state provision for birth control. Dr Wendy Greengross,

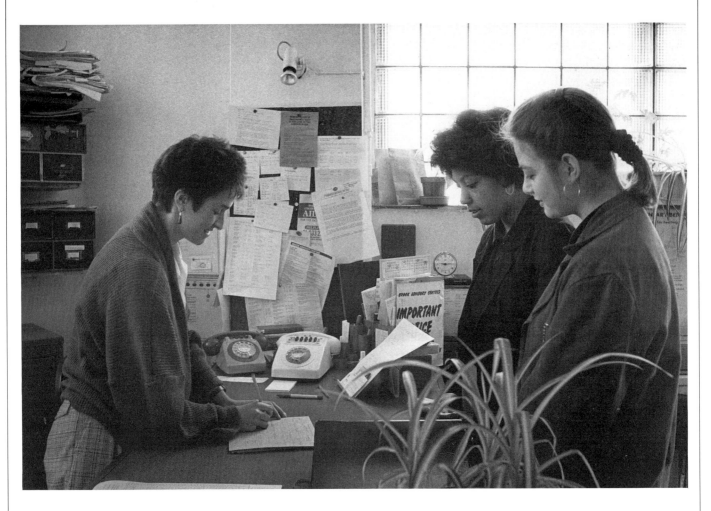

9 Girls make an appointment at a Brook Advisory Centre.

who qualified in the 1940s, remembers:

> . . . during my six years of medical training we were only
> given one half-hour's tuition on contraception. And we
> were lucky to have a registrar who would tell us anything
> at all! It was not a scheduled aspect of the syllabus. (Quoted
> in *The Compleat Woman*)

However, the Family Planning Association increased
in size and some local health authorities also ran
clinics. Birth control methods were not dependable
until the contraceptive pill was introduced in the
1960s. Contraception then became a medical matter, as
doctors had to prescribe the pill on the National
Health or by private prescription and the FPA
continued to deal with other contraceptive methods
for married women, or those within six weeks of
marriage.

There was only some unofficial advice for unmarried
women, until Helen Brook, who had worked at the

Marie Stopes clinic, left in 1964 to start the Brook
Advisory Centres with Margaret Pyke, which gave
advice to unmarried girls under 25. One of the early
Brook clients remembered:

> To be listened to, to be understood, not to be judged – this
> is where the true healing lies. ('Single Blow for Freedom',
> *The Observer*, 1989)

In 1974 free contraception for married and single
women alike was finally provided on the National
Health Service, and by 1976 the FPA had transferred
all its clinics to the NHS, retaining an information and
educational service. Brook still concentrates on the
younger age group and prefers a girl to come to a
consultation with her partner when possible.

The laws relating to abortion were also changing. In
1936 the Abortion Law Reform Association led by
Dora Russell and Stella Browne had tried to bring an
end to illegal backstreet abortions which endangered
women's lives. The law was not changed until 1967,
when an abortion could be given on health grounds if

two doctors agreed it was necessary.

Between 1969 and 1987 there have been 14 attempts in the House of Commons and two in the House of Lords to change the law on abortion. None succeeded. In 1987 to 1988 David Alton's private member's bill introduced a statutory time limit for abortion of 18 weeks, but the bill failed to go through. Since the mid-1970s the National Abortion Campaign have lobbied for 'free abortion on demand – a woman's right to choose'. Lady Helen Brook, General Manager of the London Brook Centre, believes that prevention is better than abortion.

> What Brook stands for . . . is the prevention of abortion, the prevention of the unwanted child. And the teaching of responsibility so that young people don't rush into adulthood before they are able to cope with it. (The *Guardian*, July 1989)

The general availability of information about birth control and sexual matters has greatly improved women's health and freedom today, although there are still many who are opposed to contraception or abortion on religious grounds. Controversy also continues about the age a girl should be given advice on contraception without her parents being told. Many people believe that before the age of 16 a girl is too young to receive such advice, though to deny her it could result in unwanted pregnancy.

Now in the 1990s contraceptive habits are changing again. Many doctors advise against long-term use of the pill. Claire Chilvers, a researcher for the Institute of Cancer Research, believes that women 'should aim at the lowest dose Pill for the shortest possible time', and use other contraceptive methods like the condom. The condom is also recommended to avoid infection from AIDS, which is now an increasing risk for both sexes. Dr Susie Forster, senior lecturer in venereology at St Mary's, London, says: 'A lot of the stigma has relaxed for gay men. It is the heterosexuals who are

10 Cartoonist Posy Simmonds makes fun of the new openness about contraception among the middle classes in the event of AIDs.

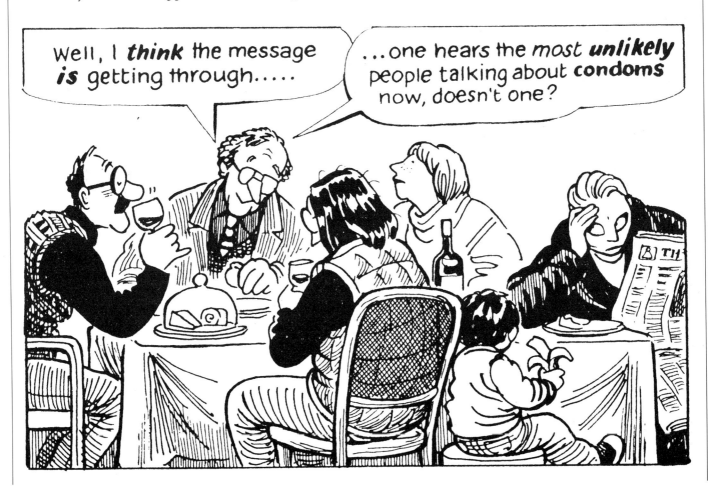

acutely aware of it now, in the same way homosexuals were four years ago' (reported in the *Guardian*, August 28 1989). Positively Women, a group directed by Caroline Guiness, has been set up to help HIV positive women, and Immunity, run by Ann Bond and David Taylor, deals with AIDS sufferers of both sexes.

The pill gave them permission to say yes; AIDS may give them permission to say no. (Wendy Thomas to the *Observer*, 1989)

Evidence

A I have had five living children and have been seven times pregnant. I belong to the working class and know only too well how bitterly the working classes need the help Dr Marie Stopes is giving . . . I thank God every day I visited the Clinic when I did . . . What do our lives become? We get broken in health, having sickly babies and too often have to go out to work to make ends meet . . . I wish Dr Marie Stopes was a multi-millionaire so, that she could open clinic in every town in England. (Letter from a patient, about 1921, quoted in Ruth Hall, *Dear Dr Stopes*)

B We knew absolutely nothing. Nothing at all. I mean, it amazes me that we didn't all get pregnant. Actually, quite a lot of the village girls did have babies, particularly with the Americans. Sex before marriage was just something that wasn't spoken about. It was all hushed up, like so much in those days. All your mother would say was, 'Be careful, whatever you do, or you'll finish up having to get married. You'll ruin your life.' (Woman who grew up in the 1940s, quoted in *You'll Never Be 16 Again*)

C Contrary to what people think we were actually using very low dose pills. We tried low doses of oestrogen, low dose progesterone, low dose of the combinations and, you know, even half got pregnant on the lowest does of one of the pills we used. So the husbands had to give their agreement. Everyone was very enthusiastic. The husbands were so pleased; one wife came back and said, 'My husband brings me flowers now'. The change from using condoms and the cap, you see. They were really delighted . . . The first symptoms we noticed were bad headaches and migraine and depression. Women began to say they stopped being interested in sex. In fact there was a joke in the early days that that was how the pill worked. (Dr Ellen Grant, who worked on clinical trials for oral contraception in the 1960s, quoted in *Out of the Doll's House*)

D The doctor in charge then asked if I'd be interested in a new male contraceptive study. I said I'd think about it and mentioned it to mates at work. They were horrified, and all said that no way would they do anything like that. But I was interested because my wife was having such awful problems with the pill. She'd put on two stone and was very miserable. I felt that if there was a genuine alternative, I'd be more than happy to use it. . . The injections themselves didn't hurt, although I did feel sore two days later. I was told it was caused by the hormone getting into the bloodstream . . . We men, who have had 30 years of not having to bother with contraception, see it as a woman's problem. I can't see men in casual relationships bothering with the injections, so I think the method will be limited to married men and those in long-term relationships. (Jimmy Bremner, who took part in a Medical Research Council trial of injections to suppress the male sperm count, quoted in the *Sunday Times*, 11 February 1990)

Questions

1 How did the unavailability of contraceptives affect women?

2 Have attitudes towards sex and contraception changed between the dates of the two women's statements in A and B? Why do you think this is so?

3 Compare the attitudes to the female pill in C and to male contraceptives in D. Should contraception be seen as a 'women's problem'?

4 Is it possible to place a fixed lower limit on the age girls can obtain advice on contraception without their parents knowing?

CHAPTER 3

Dieting

Susie Orbach (b. 1946)

The preoccupation with food is linked with a fetishizing of the female form. Women wish to acquire that elusive, eternally youthful body beautiful. (Susie Orbach, Hunger Strike)

A diet can be followed for nutritional, health or cosmetic reasons. Dieting in order to slim is generally a female pre-occupation, bound up with the present-day fashionable cult of youth and a woman's body image. When carried to extremes, relentless dieting can lead to serious eating problems – anorexia (self-starvation) and bulimia (compulsive eating, followed by self-induced vomiting). It is these extremes that concern psychotherapist Susie Orbach, whose research into women's eating problems has led her to the conclusion that they are forms of protest and must be studied in relation to the changing position of women in society.

Susie Orbach was educated at Richmond College, City University of New York, where she first met her collaborator and close friend Luise Eichenbaum in 1971. Together they helped to build up the Women's Studies BA course at the College and both were deeply committed feminists. Between 1973 and 1975 Orbach and Eichenbaum carried out research into women's psychology with the New York Feminist Therapists Study Group, in conjunction with other psycho-therapists and feminists. They opened the Women's Therapy Centre in London in 1976. The aim of the Centre was to advise women on eating problems, taking into account the social pressures specifically affecting women. Seminars, workshops and training were also part of the Centre's work. In 1981 the Women's Therapy Centre Institute for training

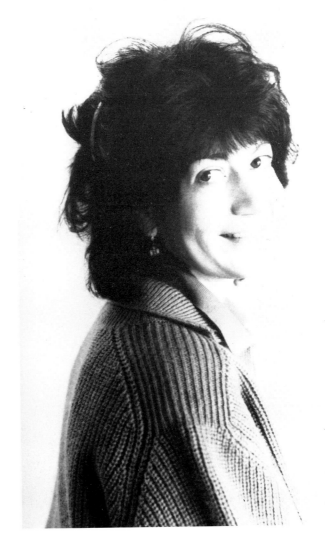

11 Psychotherapist Susie Orbach, pioneer researcher into women's eating problems.

psychotherapists opened in New York.

Susie Orbach has written several books. *Fat is a Feminist Issue* (1978) brought compulsive eating problems to the attention of the general public for the first time and suggested new methods of treatment. *Hunger Strike* (1986) was concerned with anorexia and bulimia. In collaboration with Luise Eichenbaum, she has also written *Understanding Women* and *What Do Women Want?*. Their latest book, *Bittersweet*, is about the importance of women's friendships in the modern world.

Compulsive eating was Susie Orbach's first field of research. She had herself gone through the experience of dieting, followed by bouts of compulsive eating, and the self-hatred that accompanied it. Although people of either gender can be fat, compulsive eating and the problems that go with it are almost entirely suffered by women.

The problems have also become much more acute over the past 20 years – a period which has coincided with radical changes in women's place in society. During these years advertising and the media have also started influencing every aspect of life, and it is difficult to avoid images of the so-called 'ideal woman'.

Ms Orbach saw that there were many complex reasons why women became fat, one being that it was a way of avoiding 'society's sex stereotypes'. The aim of her therapy is to discover the emotional motivation behind the desire to eat. Some women who became fat believed they would be judged on their personalities rather than their bodies. Also, in an attempt at self-assertion, they felt that their larger size would give them a more forceful physical presence and would

12 This late nineteenth-century cartoon makes fun of the new bride's attempts at cooking.

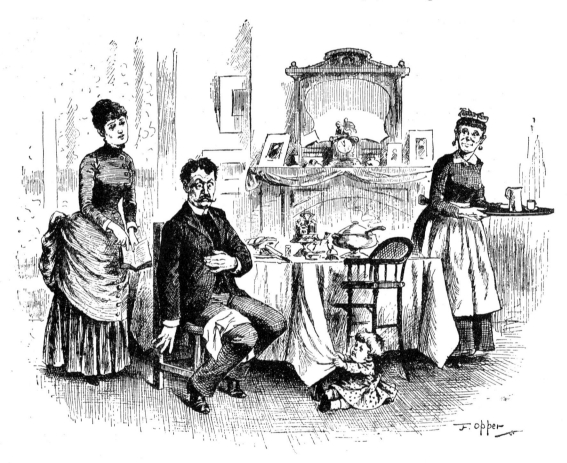

THE AGE OF HANDBOOKS.—No. II.

" I think you are perfectly horrid to find fault with the dinner, Henry ; I got it all out of the ' Young Housekeeper's Infallible Cookery-Book,' and it ought to be good, I'm sure."

make people take them seriously.

Ms Orbach carried her arguments a stage further in *Hunger Strike*. In a series of case studies of anorectic teenage girls, she suggested that anorexia nervosa rises partly from the adolescent's anxiety about growing up.

> We saw how in Jean's case the physical event of her menstruation caused an alarm and resulted in her becoming fearful of what her body could do independently. Her response was to mould and control that body as best she could. (*Hunger Strike*)

In a society with increasing pressures on women to be successful at work and to run a home at the same time, many women feel their bodies are the one area they can control.

Many women also have the feeling that they can never measure up to the female ideal of the day, constantly reiterated in newspapers, magazines and advertising, that to be thin is to be sexually desirable. The female identification with food and cooking also causes conflicting pressures. On the one hand women are expected to prepare meals – feminity and food are linked with love in many people's minds – but if women are to remain slim, they cannot eat much. Another source of tension is the relationship between mother and daughter, as mothers sometimes resent the

new freedoms enjoyed by their daughters. By rejecting food a woman is in effect on hunger strike – against these intolerable pressures.

Therapy at the Centres includes discussions on personal and family history, the eating habits of parents and the various routines and the rituals that those suffering from anorexia and bulimia follow. Whereas medical treatment usually involves hospitalization and forced feeding, Ms Orbach believes in making her clients responsible for their actions, after first understanding their underlying motives for dieting.

Susie Orbach has now left the Women's Therapy Centre in London, but has retained an active interest in the project. Although today the Centre covers a wide range of female psychological problems, nearly one quarter of the enquiries are about eating disorders. From this the Centre concludes:

> . . . food is a dominating focus in women's lives . . . Relating obsessively to food becomes a means whereby women's emotional needs and anxieties are expressed . . . hardly a single woman feels happy about her bodyshape or size, and many women experience a constant sense of failure in not being able to live up to society's image of the 'ideal woman'.

Questions

1 Why does advertising have a dangerous effect on many women?
2 Does becoming fat or anorectic help a woman to avoid 'society's sex stereotypes'?
3 Are women's eating disorders more effectively treated by psychotherapy than by traditional medicine?

Diet and Nutrition

Paintings and statues from the past show how the ideals of feminine beauty have changed throughout history. Fat women were admired in primitive societies, as fatness signified fertility. The Venus de Milo would be a size 16 today and Rubens' women were definitely outsize.

Ever since the 1920s and the beginnings of female emancipation, women have been expected to be slim. Since the 1960s, the ideal typified by models like

Twiggy has been verging on the anorectic. The emphasis has been on youth, and in recent years there has been a disturbing trend of casting teenage movie stars like Brooke Shields and Jodie Foster in highly sexual roles. Although the ideal feminine shape today is more like that of a 14-year-old girl, in fact most women are size 14 or over.

> I suppose you really do believe that your happiness is consequent on your size? That an inch or two one way or

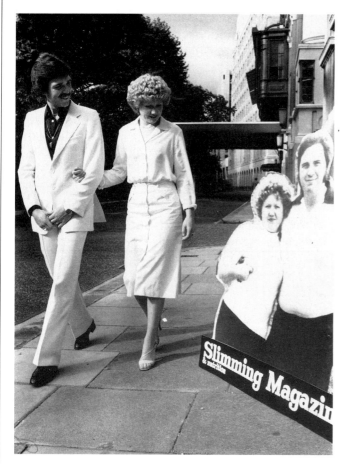

13 This couple have just received first prize from Slimming Magazine *for losing eleven stone between them.*

the other would make you truly loved? Equating prettiness with sexuality, and sexuality with happiness? It is a very debased view of sexuality you take . . . (Fay Weldon; *The Fat Woman's Joke*)

Although both sexes are now figure conscious, women are more likely to carry dieting to obsessive extremes. Anorexia was first named in the nineteenth century by the physician W.W. Gull. Then, as now, it was a disguised cry for help, similar to those signs of emotional distress (fainting fits and hysteria) familiar in Victorian novels. A great many Victorian girls felt imprisoned in the female role of the day, Florence Nightingale and Elizabeth Barrett Browning among them, and obtained freedom of a kind through ill-health.

The Victorians stressed the importance of a slim figure, small waist and upright posture, but by the end of the century the ideal figure was larger. Madame Bayard, advertising various creams and potions of her own invention, wrote:

Ladies who wish to become plump without being stout, and have a complexion like milk and roses, cannot do better than drink the new tea that is now all the rage in Paris, I mean 'Serkys' – which can be had at this office. (*Toilet Hints or How to Preserve Beauty, and How to Acquire It*, quoted in *Beauty In History*)

The influence of professional models on the way women wanted to look did not have much effect until after the First World War, when films and photography helped to spread fashions, which at that time favoured a slim, liberated, boyish figure – an image which has remained. During the last 40 years, television and advertising have had an even stronger impact on clothes and body image. Twiggy, the model whose extreme slimness influenced women's fashion in the 1960s, was only 15 when she was first spotted by Justin de Villeneuve. She weighed six and a half stone (41 kilos), and car stickers carried the motto: 'Forget

14 An Edwardian postcard ridiculing fat women.

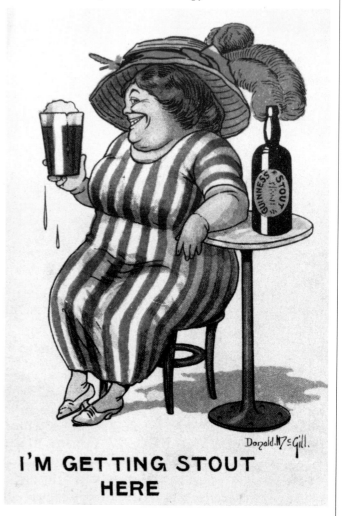

I'M GETTING STOUT HERE

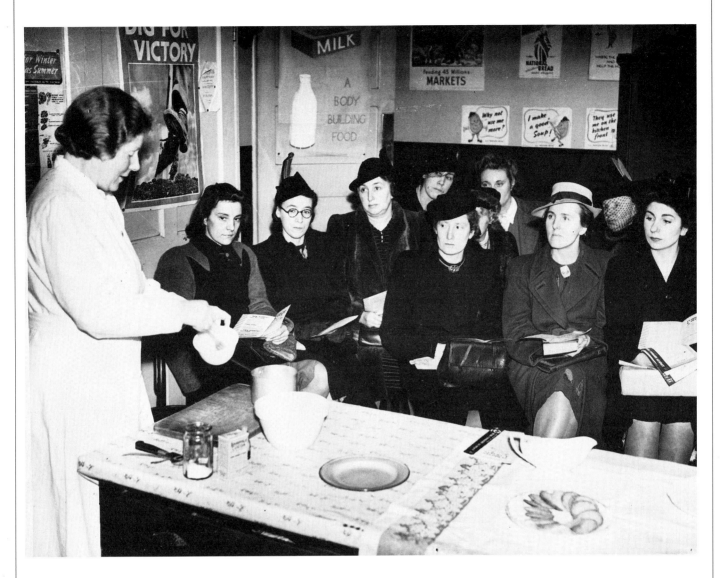

15 A Ministry of Food cookery demonstration in the outpatients department of the Soho Hospital for Women in 1943.

Oxfam. Feed Twiggy'.

Fatness is presented by the media as being the antithesis of everything that is desirable and efficient. Although too much weight is bad for a person's health, part of Susie Orbach's work has been to get women to accept the figures that they have been born with and not to try to achieve unrealistic impossibilities by diet. In recent years the Women's Liberation Movement has done much to challenge the physical patterns imposed on women.

Spare Rib was one of the first journals to look into eating disorders, and Susie Orbach contributed articles. Various self-help groups, like the Spare Tyre Theatre Company, have also taken up the cause of Fat Liberation – the acceptance of fat people as they are, not as the sufferers of some medical abnormality. A representative of the London Fat Women's Group,

speaking on television in 1989, spoke of the discrimination against them in jobs, their lack of choice in clothes and the fact that people always assumed they were greedy.

> I also object to the word 'obesity' . . . It's a doctor's word – used to classify us as a 'medical problem' and to justify their abuse of us. Fat is what we are and it's what we've reclaimed both the word and the right to be fat. (Letter in *Spare Rib*, 1985)

Dieting is almost entirely a twentieth-century phenomenon and is restricted to the Western world. Although there were a number of diet regimes published in the twenties and thirties, slimming really became big business in the late 1960s with endless

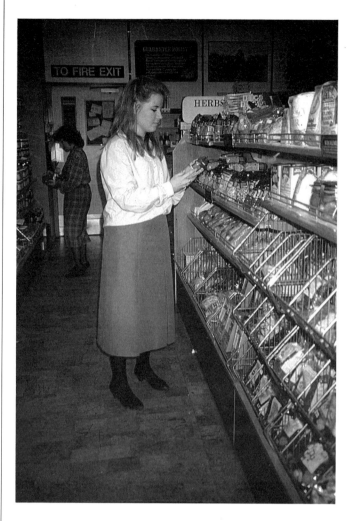

16 A woman buys groceries in a modern health food shop.

with a balanced diet. Women have always done the cooking and shopping, although men have traditionally been chefs. In working-class rural communities in the past men ate better than women, who got smaller portions and not so much meat.

> The remark was constantly made to me that 'the husband wins the bread, and must have the best food'. (Dr Edward Smith, 1863, quoted in *A History of Women's Bodies*)

Upper-class women had more opportunity to consider the art of cooking and many kept books of their own recipes. By the seventeenth and eighteenth centuries some had started to publish cookery books – among them Eliza Smith, Hannah Glasse and Sarah Phillips. Some of the nineteenth-century cookery books are still famous today, for example, Elizabeth Acton's *Modern Cookery For Private Families* (1845), Mrs Beeton's *Book of Household Management* (1861) and *The Boston Cooking-School Cook Book* (1896) by Fannie Farmer, an American writer who introduced a precise method of measuring ingredients.

Nutrition did not become a serious concern until the beginning of the twentieth century, when the importance of vitamins was discovered. During the First World War soldiers fighting the Gallipoli Campaign were found to have scurvy, after which research into nutrition began at the Lister Institute in London. Two women, Harriette Chick and Margaret Hume carried out pioneer work while most of the male staff of the institute were away in the army. After the war Ms Chick headed a team of scientists who went to Vienna to study the effects of severe malnutrition.

Research was given a new impetus during the Second World War, when the government established the basic nutritional requirements on which food rationing was founded. Among the scientists working for the Ministry of Food were Harriet Chick and Margaret Hume at the Lister Institute, Elsie Widdowson at the Department of Experimental Medicine, Cambridge, and Dorothy Hollingsworth based with the Ministry.

Most people were better fed during the Second World War than in the previous 20 years. This was because rationing gave everyone equal rights to basic foods, which were cheaper because of a government subsidy. The Ministry of Food recruited mainly female lecturers and demonstrators to help improve the nation's diet. The most famous of these was Marguerite Patten, whose recipes and advice encouraged women to cook healthy, balanced meals

books, pamphlets and magazines on the subject, self-help groups like Weight Watchers and expensive health farms. A survey conducted by the Royal College of Physicians in 1983 reported that, at any one time, 65 per cent of British women were on a diet. Much of the emphasis is now on health rather than slimming and includes a new enthusiasm for exercise – also sometimes carried to excess, as dieting can be. Jane Fonda, film star and pioneer of aerobics, has confessed that she suffered from anorexia and bulimia for ten years and also took drugs to lose weight. 'Nor did any doctor warn us that we could become addicted to them – as I did'.

Ironically, while pressure is put on women by the media to achieve a slim figure, they are the ones traditionally responsible for providing their families with the limited wartime rations. Her influence continued long after the war with her many radio and television appearances and her cookery books, of which there are over 155.

Nutritional research into vitamins continued after the war, and by the 1960s problems of dietary intolerance were being explored. Women today play a major part in maintaining nutritional standards. Among them are recipe writers like Elizabeth David, founders of self-help groups like Maryon Stewart (*The Women's Nutritional Advisory Service*), Amelia Nathan Hill (*Action Against Allergy*), Sally Bunday and Irene Colquhoun (*The Hyperactive Children's Support Group*) and Margery Hall (*Sanity*) – who campaigns for research into the biochemical factors leading to mental illness. In recent years women's magazines have helped to spread information about healthy eating and we are probably better informed than we have ever been on the nutritional content of different foodstuffs.

Evidence

A Women of all ages, especially expectant and nursing mothers, stand in special need of not merely ample but correct food and it is precisely the correct foods that they find it most difficult to afford within the family budget. As often as not the mother keeps herself short of proper nourishment in her efforts to provide the maximum for her menfolk and growing children. (Catherine Carswell, writing in the *Manchester Guardian* in the 1930s, quoted in *Women Talking*)

B I've only dieted once in my life, when I got married; I went down from size 20 to size 12 in five months and I was utterly unhappy. I regained the weight pretty quickly and never felt tempted to try to stick at an intermediate level. My family is short and plump, so I must have a slower metabolism than other people. People tend to stereotype you as a fat slob if you're my size, but I actually lead a pretty active life. . . Interviewers often describe me to my face as 'rotund', 'ample' or 'happy' – never fat or big – and that's more offensive. They want to know how I 'cope' with my size, as though it were some terrible physical disability; I feel like asking them how *they* cope with their sagging knees or whatever. (Dawn French, the comedian, talks to Anthea Gerrie in the *Sunday Times*, 11 February 1990)

C Deep down bulimic women aren't merely afraid of getting fat (although they don't want to be); they are unsure about how to relate to their feelings, their upsets, their aspirations, their wish for independence, and their shame about feeling needy and dependent. It is their emotional lives that frighten and repel them . . . it is possible to find ways out of this tortuous and secret cycle of bingeing and expelling. A good place to start is to tell a friend, a counsellor, a sister – someone who won't judge but will lend a sympathetic ear. Be patient, compassionate and caring with yourself . . . recognise that you are in trouble and that you need to look after yourself. (Psychotherapist Susie Orbach; *ELLE* report, 'A Private Dysfunction)

D I have been a vegan for nearly a year now, and before that I was a vegetarian for three years. My reasons for giving up meat and fish were based on the argument that it is wasteful to graze animals on land which could be used to produce cereals and vegetables, and that the seas are over-fished. I was not concerned at all about the way in which animals are treated, but when I stopped eating them my awareness in this direction increased. So when I gave up eating animal products it was out of disgust at methods of egg and milk production . . . I think it's important to question things we take for granted and what we should eat to stay healthy is rarely looked at critically. (Jenny Muir, *Spare Rib*, November 1984)

Questions

1 Why did women deprive themselves of food in the past? Does this still happen today? If so, is it for the same reasons?

2 What does Dawn French (B) object to about the words interviewers use to describe her? How can the language used to describe women help support the sex stereotypes in our society?

3 How many different attitudes to food and weight are expressed in these sources? Why is food a 'dominating focus in women's lives'?

CHAPTER 4

Environment

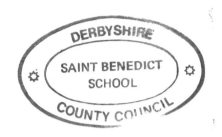

Rachel Carson (1907–64)

The history of life on earth has been a history of interaction between living things and their surroundings . . . only within the moment of time represented by the present century has one species – man – acquired significant power to alter the nature of his world. (Rachel Carson, *The Silent Spring*)

Rachel Carson was one of the first to alert people to the fact that scientific progress had serious disadvantages, as industrial and chemical pollution were poisoning the planet with increasing rapidity. She questioned the right of anybody to upset the balance of nature, however admirable their motives might be. She started her crusade soon after the Second World War, when advances in the chemical industry stimulated by the war, seemed to point the way to more efficient crop production through the use of chemical fertilizers and pesticides.

Ms Carson came from a farming family living in Springdale, USA. She was educated at Pennsylvania College for Women and Johns Hopkins University. Although always interested in writing, she studied natural history, becoming genetic biologist for the American Fish and Wildlife Service from 1936 until 1949 and Editor in Chief in 1949.

While researching into offshore life at Words Hole Oceanographic Institute, Rachel Carson became interested in ecology. Her first books were about marine biology – *Under The Sea Wind* in 1941, followed by *The Sea Around Us* in 1951 which became a world-wide best seller. The book told how the seas were formed and the way in which life emerged, going on to describe the teeming life of the sea in all its variety.

At the time the book was published there was increasing interest in the natural world. Rachel Carson's sense of wonder in the natural world and her knowledge of the interdependence of living creatures made her realize that humans might be endangering the delicate balance of life with pollutants.

After another book about marine biology, *The Edge of the Sea* (1955), Rachel Carson expressed her fears in *The Silent Spring* (1962), a controversial work which exposed dangers to the environment caused by the indiscriminate use of herbicides, insecticides and pesticides. She forecast a future where insects and the birds which fed on them would be wiped out, and asked the question:

. . . Who has decided – who has the right to decide – for the countless legions of people who were not consulted that the supreme value is a world without insects, even though it be also a sterile world ungraced by the curving wing of a bird in flight? (*The Silent Spring*)

The fifties and sixties were times of technological progress when people were finding chemicals the quick solution to problems in the home and in industry, as well as in agriculture. Chemical fertilizers and pesticides appeared to be an answer to the world food shortage, and indeed, between 1945 and 1975 world food production doubled. Only now are the long-term side-effects becoming apparent.

Ms Carson's opinions were much ahead of her time and her book was attacked because of business interests, but it was received enthusiastically by the general public. Pollution problems were not yet as bad

26

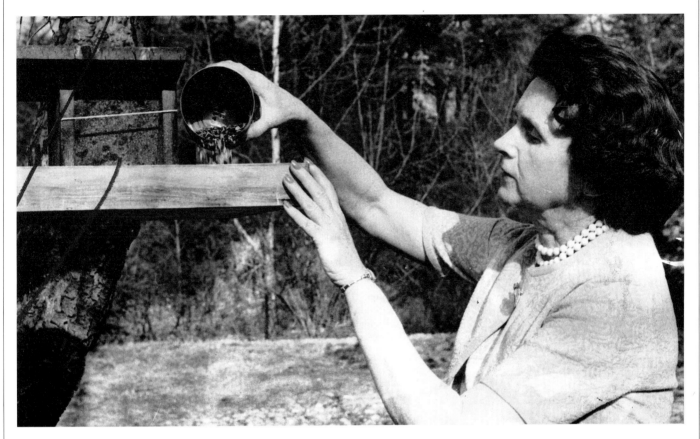

17 Conservationist Rachel Carson in 1964.

in Britain as they were in the USA but it was clear that the situation was getting worse. Thousands of non-selective chemicals were on sale which had the power to kill every living insect. Ms Carson asked:

> Can anyone believe it is possible to lay down such a barrage of poisons on the surface of the earth without making it unfit for all life? They should not be called 'insecticides' but 'biocides'. (*The Silent Spring*)

The pesticide DDT, which had been developed as a chemical weapon during the war, was the main culprit attacked in *The Silent Spring*. Ms Carson pointed out that it was one of the most environmentally dangerous of the agrochemicals, because it was passed on from one organism to another through the food chain and stored for long periods in the body fat of animals. Ultimately, many birds and small mammals could be wiped out because of the build-up of the chemical.

A 'silent spring' had already become a reality in parts of the USA as many birds were dying. The environment would not only be less beautiful when herbicides had destroyed the wild flowers but there would be repercussions on all forms of life. Indiscriminate spraying with chemicals also harmed the soil and polluted rivers and the sea. Humans, too, would suffer, and Ms Carson collected evidence of links with cancer, liver diseases and nerve end damage.

> As man proceeds towards his announced goal of the conquest of nature, he has written a depressing record of destruction, directed not only against the earth he inhabits but against the life that shares it with him. (*The Silent Spring*)

After a public outcry following the publication of Rachel Carson's book, many countries forbad the use of DDT and other pesticides that could harm wildlife. DDT was not banned in Britain until 1984 and it is still used illegally today. Rachel Carson received many awards for her scientific and literary achievements, which included the Literary Award for the Council of Women of the USA (1956), the Schwatzer Prize for Animal Welfare (1963) and the Conservationist of the Year Award of the National Wildlife Federation (1963). She was in poor health for the last few years of her life and ironically died of cancer. Concern for the environment, particularly among the young, dates from *The Silent Spring*.

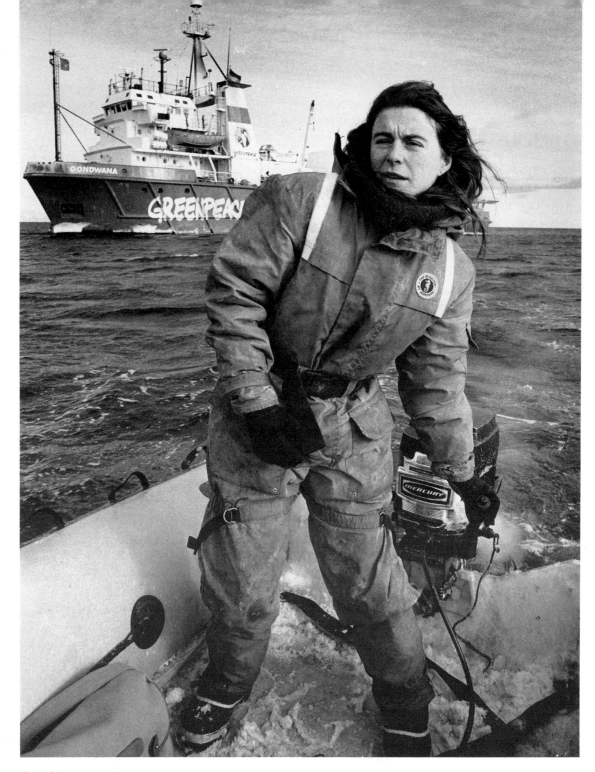

18 A member of the Greenpeace expedition campaigning against the dumping of toxic wastes in Antarctica, 1988/9.

Questions

1 How did Rachel Carson become concerned about the environment?
2 Why did it take so long for people to realize the harmful effects of chemical pollutants on the environment?
3 How can environmental pollution affect human health?

Pollutants and Health

Although the Green revolution and feminism do not necessarily go together, today women in many countries are campaigning to improve the environment, particularly when they feel that their children's health is in danger. There have been many examples in the past of women's concern with ecology. In the eighteenth century Mary Wollstonecraft forecast a time when the earth would be over-farmed and there would be famine. In the nineteenth century many of the pioneer feminists belonged to the anti-vivisection movement. Ynestra King, an American 'eco-feminist', believes that it is dangerous to say that women are 'closer to Nature', as this could lead to the assumption that a woman's role is passive. She does, however, concede that women are natural conservationists:

> It's a way of being, which understands that there are connections between all living things and that indeed we women are the fact and the flesh of connectedness. (Quoted in Stephenie Leyland & Leonie Caldecott, *Reclaim the Earth*, Womens Press, 1983)

Jonathon Porritt, former Director of Friends of the Earth, also thinks women have a special influence on environmental issues:

> I don't think one is being sexist here. There is a higher awareness in women of these issues: the polls have shown this. Women are the ones who have helped to change consumer patterns, and that is very important. Women do think more about the future, and the impact of things on the environment – which is why their contribution is so critical. (Quoted in *Women's Journal*, November 1988)

The health of all living creatures is dependent on the air they breathe and the food they eat. Although nuclear power helps to conserve other dwindling sources of energy, women are particularly concerned that radiation fall-out of the kind suffered at Chernobyl in 1986, should not harm the health of their babies and children.

Women have had close links with the Peace Movement since the time of the suffragettes. In the 1950s leaders like Pat Arrowsmith campaigned for

19 Women protest against the nuclear arms race and the threat to the environment.

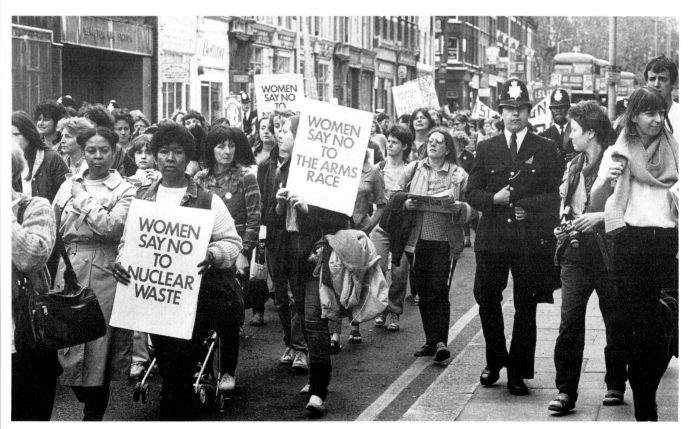

nuclear disarmament and in the 1980s the Greenham Common women protested for many years against the American Cruise missile base. This concern now extends to peaceful uses of nuclear power, and CND is active in the Green movement. Linda Churnside, Chair of Green CND, says: 'Practically every women in CND has been to Greenham at some time and they've been a big influence'.

A report on the nuclear fuel plant at Sellafield, published in February 1990, has found that children born to male employees have a higher than average risk of contracting cancer, if the father worked in radio-active areas during the six months before the baby was conceived. According to Dr Janet Tawn, who was in charge of the investigatory team, these men showed chromosome abnormalities four to six times higher than those who worked outside the plant. Hilda Murrell's campaign against all uses of nuclear power may have caused her death in 1984.

Environmental problems are global, rather than national. The air is polluted by factory smoke, car exhaust fumes and other gadgets of modern life, causing respiratory diseases and lung cancer. Airborne lead poisoning can cause kidney or nerve disease and lead ultimately to permanent brain damage in young children. Toxic waste discharged into rivers and seas contaminates fish and the poisons are passed on to humans, giving rise to illnesses of the brain and nervous system.

There was an outcry in 1988 when a shipment of PCB chemical waste was brought by sea to Britain for disposal. PCBs, like DDT which Rachel Carson opposed, only break down very slowly in the environment. In use since 1929, there are traces of PCBs everywhere, even in our own bodies. Women's breast milk may now contain these dangerous chemicals, according to a German survey conducted in 1981.

Acid rain, caused by burning fossil fuel in Britain and West Germany, falls on Swedish soil, damaging wildlife, killing trees and disfiguring buildings. The destruction of rain forests in Central America results in climatic changes, the death of wild life, soil erosion and loss of livelihood for the inhabitants. In her study *In the Rain Forest*, Catherine Caufield has collected statistics to show what the world will lose if the forests are destroyed. Organizations like Friends of the Earth and Greenpeace campaign against these abuses of the natural world.

Recently we have been made aware of a dangerous reduction in the ozone level (the band of gases surrounding the Earth). The gap discovered in the ozone layer in Antarctica means there is a greater risk of ultraviolet radiation, which produces skin cancer. We are advised to stop using products containing chlorofluorocarbons (man-made chemicals), most commonly found in aerosols, fridges, air-conditioning plants, dry cleaning solvents and plastic foam. Women, who are the prime users of aerosols, are helping to ban their use, and the campaign has been encouraged by women's magazines. In 1987 Fay Weldon wrote a play about the ozone layer, *The Hole in the Top of the World*. She said to Jonathon Porritt:

> A couple of years ago, if you talked about what was happening to the ozone layer, most people thought you were making it up. Now they know it's true . . . The pace of environmental destruction which now threatens our lives and health has become much more extreme, so art will reflect this . . . (Quoted in *The Coming of the Greens*)

One of the most influential women in the study of world environment is Ms Gro Harlem Brundtland, Prime Minister of Norway. She chaired the World Commission on Environment and Development in 1983 which produced the report *Our Common Future*. The report studied the potential dangers to the environment arising from individual countries' industrial expansion, and recommended 'sustainable development', a theory first put forward in the 1960s by Barbara Ward, one of the founders of the International Institute for Environment and Development.

The last few years have also seen the rise of 'eco-feminism' in the developing world, where women are directly involved with industrialized agriculture and fully aware of its destructive effects on health. The most striking example has been the Chipko Movement in northern India, 1973, where women protested against the destruction of the forest – which provided their livelihood – by logging companies. As director of Friends of the Earth in Malaysia, Chee Yok Ling campaigns against the use of the chemical paraquat (a quick-acting herbicide) on rubber plantations, as it endangers the health of women who use the sprays and that of their unborn children.

Vandana Shiva is director of the Research Foundation for Science, Technology and Natural Resource Policy at Dehradun in northern India. She left her job as a physicist for ideological reasons, and said of her decision, 'the reaction of nuclear systems

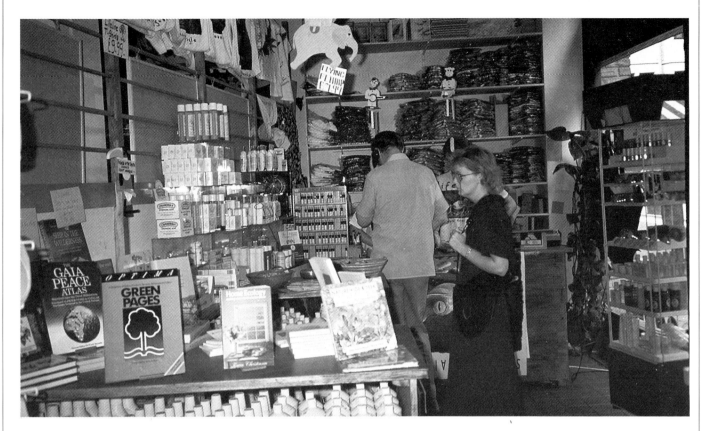

20 A shop selling ecologically sound products.

with living systems is being kept from the people' (interview in the *Observer*, March 1989). She believes that rural Indian workers are the best environmental managers in her country and is in favour of 'appropriate development' rather than scientific industrialization of the land.

Some Green societies for women only have been started during the last few years. The Women's Environmental Network began in 1987 and its present director is Bernadette Vallely. The founders, who include Anita Roddick of the Body Shop and the Labour MP Joan Ruddock, believe that:

> As major consumers, women are in a position of power to influence and control the destruction and exploitation of the environment. Women need to be in the forefront of the struggle for the environment with our unique experiences and visions of the future and our logical, caring perspective which has too often been ignored and undermined.

There is growing opposition to factory farming and the use of animals for experimentation. Support is increasing for campaigns to protect species which face extinction because parts of their bodies are used in various products. In Britain the cosmetic industry is now coming round to a Green attitude, largely because of lobbying from women. Pioneers in the use of ecologically sound products, produced without cruelty to animals, are Martha Hill, Helen Ambrosen (Cosmetics to Go) and Anita Roddick (The Body Shop).

> Animals should not suffer in laboratory tests for our vanity. Whales should not be slaughtered to provide moisture creams. Placenta is unacceptable as a cosmetic ingredient. Aerosols should not be used as they are indisposable . . . Packaging should not be wasteful or unnecessarily expensive. (Anita Roddick, *The Body Shop Book*)

The invention of non-biodegradable substances like plastic, coupled with an increase in packaging mean that waste-disposal problems have also increased. Women everywhere help to organize recycling of household materials or run information services, like Valerie Elliott at the Centre for Environmental Information (opened in 1986). In politics, Sara Parkin is International Secretary of the UK Green Party.

Women are involved in the protection of the environment at many different levels in Britain today. Some are novelists like Fay Weldon and Doris Lessing, others are journalists on national newspapers or write on

Green topics for women's magazines. Photographers such as Fay Godwin draw attention to threatened areas of the countryside, and editor Liz Rigbey raises ecological issues in the radio programme *The Archers*. The cartoonist Posy Simmonds pokes fun at the middle-class aspect of the Green philosophy. She thinks that:

a lot of greening comes from women. They're usually the ones who care about health, and food and nurturing. They're the ones who tell stories to their children and have to answer all those difficult philosophical questions like 'What happens to bunnies when they die?' (Quoted in *The Coming of the Greens*)

Evidence

A So we started to cut the wire to bring to the attention of the public the wall of secrecy and lies around Sellafield. I was around and had young children when the big fire happened in 1957. Over the years there have been more accidents and leaks. About 100 women went to mark the fire and the six babies who died around there that year. The gates were very securely closed. It looked so very strong and inaccessible. But I was walking around a bit and realised that no matter how strong the gates were, underneath the fence was just soil. So I started to scrape it away, just with sticks, and then we got under it. (Catharina Barnes, a 72-year-old former nurse, quoted in the *Guardian*, March 30 1989)

B In her unit for Environmental Medicine at London's Lister Hospital, Dr Monro has seen hundreds of terrible instances of the disabling and generalized damage which food and chemical sensitivities are now responsible for . . . Massive environmental pollution renders us all vulnerable . . . Perhaps it will be generally accepted one day that the rise in chronic disease at all ages, the frightening vulnerability of our young to addictive habits like smoking, drinking and drug-taking, the learning disorders which are now so common, the behavioural problems and hooliganism which turn classrooms into battlegrounds, and the escalating violence in our Western society which baffles sociologists and politicians alike, are at least in part the result of this genetic damage. (Barbara Griggs, *The Food Factor*)

C Being green probably started with my mother. She hated wasting anything. She never chucked out food, paper bags, jars

or anything else she could find a use for. I think a lot of women used to live that way. My mum brought us up with a knowledge of and sensitivity to the natural world around us . . . It taught me that humans are one tiny interrelated facet of a world in which every human blunder has an extraordinarily distorting effect throughout the world and throughout time. If more people understood that, then a lot of destruction that's going on in the world wouldn't be happening. People seem to think other living things exist purely so that we can exploit them. But I want to live not just in relation to people, but as a part of the *whole* of nature. (Film star Julie Christie, quoted in Jonathon Porritt & David Winner, *The Coming of the Greens*)

D We didn't come into the business saying we're going to be environmentally sensitive and concerned. Business ideas don't work like that. I was simply in love with the idea of setting up a small shop and selling natural products. I was fascinated by the ingredients, which came from tropical areas . . . Certain things cleansed, polished and protected the skin without having to be formulated into a cream or shampoo. They worked brilliantly and they had been doing so for more than 2,000 years. The environmental thing came out of other values. I had been involved in things like CND, Freedom From Hunger and Shelter, which were all about humanitarian issues. The question of why things in the environment were so screwed up never really occurred to me until I met the people affected. (Anita Roddick, founder and managing director of The Body Shop, quoted in *The Coming of the Greens*)

Questions

1 Why was Catharina Barnes making a protest at Sellafield (A)? What other protests of this kind have there been?

2 What effects of environmental pollution on human health are mentioned in B? Can you think of any recent outbreaks of illness which have been at least partly caused by modern technology?

3 Why do you think women have been among the most committed campaigners on environmental issues? Is it sexist to say that they are natural conservationists?

CHAPTER 5

Exercise

Prunella Stack (b. 1914)

Women should take themselves in hand and learn to prevent their ailments, not only by relying on medical cures, but on their own powers of positive health. (Mary Bagot Stack)

Prunella Stack was born at the outbreak of the First World War and her father was killed in action in 1917. Her mother Mary (Mollie) Stack had, before her marriage, studied the physical training methods of Mrs Josef Conn, who was pioneering new exercise techniques for women in Paris. The exercises were based on posture and balance, linked with breathing control. Mrs Stack returned to her career as a tutor of the method after her husband's death and started private exercise classes for women and children.

The need for sport and physical training for girls was first recognized towards the end of the nineteenth century, largely by the pioneers of women's education. Before this the only exercise taught in schools had been drill, which was designed mainly for boys to instil discipline. Educationists like Miss Buss and Miss Beale believed in the importance of good posture and graceful movement for girls. As the new schools for girls were modelled on boys' public schools, games also became part of the curriculum.

Among the early advocates of exercise for women were Madame Osterburg, who taught the Swedish Ling system of physical training, and Isadora Duncan, who pioneered natural movement in dance. Ruby Ginner and Margaret Morris taught variations of Isadora Duncan's 'Greek Dancing' movements to music. Mary Stack evolved her own exercises which incorporated dance and music, believing that the 'body of health' which she trained should lead to the 'body of expression'.

Little do we realise the delight that awaits us when we have trained the body to be its own instrument within the great orchestra of Life . . . This cannot be done until in each one inner harmony exists, a rhythmic balance of body and spirit. Scientific training of the body along these high standards was carried out successfully by the Greeks, but then the standards were set by men. Women are the natural race builders of the world. It is they who should be responsible for its physique. (Mary Bagot Stack, *Building the Body Beautiful*)

In 1925 Mrs Stack gave her first demonstration of exercise and dance at the Aeolian Hall in London and in 1925 she opened a training school, later known as the Bagot Stack Health School. 'Greek Dancing' was an important part of the curriculum, and her daughter Prunella helped to publicize the exercises, taking part in displays and being photographed by the press. In 1930 Prunella qualified as a teacher at the school, and in 1931 Mary Stack published *Building the Body Beautiful*, describing her work.

The Women's League of Health and Beauty was founded in 1930 as Mary Stack wanted to hold classes for working girls at prices they could afford. The YMCA, London, provided the first premises, and pupils were charged 2s 6d to join. Girls were expected to buy a badge at 2s and wore white blouses and black satin pants. Publicity demonstrations in Hyde Park brought in more members and by 1933 the League was thriving and had its own magazine *Mother and Daughter*. Trained teachers from the Bagot Stack Health School held classes and advised on diet and

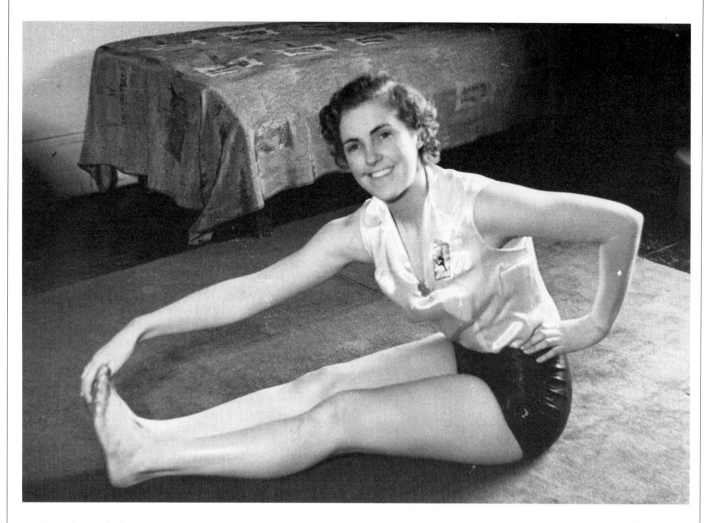

21 Prunella Stack demonstrates an exercise in the 1930s.

hygiene. Classes quickly became popular, as they gave women young and old the chance to get away from home into a club atmosphere. The League was fun and good for you as well. Similar exercise classes like Keep-Fit were soon started.

Prunella Stack took part in all the League's big events and at the death of her mother in 1935 took on the leadership. Although the League was very successful by this time, it was regarded with some suspicion by the orthodox teachers of physical education. By the end of 1935 there were branches in Australia, Hong Kong, Canada and Eire, and 64 new centres had also opened in England. In 1936, when membership was approaching 100,000, the League was asked to join the new Central Council of Recreative Physical Training. The following year Prunella Stack joined the Fitness Council, formed by the government to improve the nation's health. The Prime Minister Stanley Baldwin wrote to her:

As you are no doubt aware, the Government have already announced in general terms their intention of supplementing measures for the improvement of the National physique. They have particularly in mind the need for providing increased facilities and opportunities for physical training and recreation for young people who have left school. I do not think it is going too far to say that the success of the Scheme may well depend on the suitability of the personnel of the council, and I tender to you a very cordial invitation to serve as a member . . .

Prunella Stack continued to work tirelessly for the League until war broke out and their activities were curtailed for the duration, as many of the members were doing war work. In 1938 she married David Douglas-Hamilton, who died on active service. The Bagot Stack Health School re-opened in 1946 and the first peacetime rally and display took place.

Through the personal dedication of Prunella Stack the League has survived up to the present day, although there is now a good deal of competition from other forms of exercise like aerobics. The Bagot Stack teacher training course moved from the old premises to Morley College shortly after the war, keeping the name and independent control. Prunella was Principal of the college from 1957 to 1961. The course closed in 1970, as a full-time two-year training course was no longer viable. In future there was to be part-time regional training, and a government subsidy – in the old days the College had been self-supporting.

Today, there are branches of the League all over the world and the membership covers all ages. In 1986 Prunella Stack started a new section for women in their teens and twenties called STYLE (Stretching, Toning, Young, Lively Exercise) to adapt to competition from new youth-orientated exercise classes like those run by Pineapple. There is also now a branch for the elderly and disabled called EXTEND. The League is now known as Health and Beauty Exercise and members wear a V-necked leotard.

Questions

1 What were Mary Bagot Stack's reasons for setting up an exercise and dance school?

2 What alternative forms of exercise existed for women before the Bagot Stack Health School?

3 Why do you think Prunella Stack's form of exercise is still popular with women today?

Sport – The Emancipator

For women . . . beauty of face and form is one of the chief essentials, but unlimited indulgence in violent outdoor sports . . . cannot have but an unwomanly effect on a young girl's mind no less than on her appearance . . . let them leave rough outdoor pastimes to those for whom they are naturally intended – men. (*Badminton Magazine*, early 1900s)

The Women's League of Health and Beauty was only one of the ways in which women found health and liberation through exercise. In the Victorian age women were supposed to be delicate, passive and ladylike, debarred from strenuous exercise because it might impair their capacity to have children or make them less feminine. Although there was a tremendous enthusiasm for sport in the boys' public schools in the early nineteenth century, exercise was strictly for men only.

By the mid-nineteenth century, women who were campaigning for equal education were also questioning their exclusion from sport.

The usual and purely arbitrary notion of only certain games and certain bodily motions being decorous for the female sex is a miserable restriction on the 'individuality' of the individual. (Bessie Rayner Parkes, *Remarks on the Education of Girls*, 1854: quoted in *Sport and the Physical Emancipation of English Women*)

The pioneers of physical education for women approached the problem on four different fronts – gymnastics, sports, athletics and dancing. In the Victorian period, dancing was one of the few ways a woman could get exercise, and it was not until the early years of the twentieth century that Isadora Duncan's free-expression methods, known as 'Greek Dancing', became popular. Apart from dancing, the only exercise classes taught in girls' schools were 'callisthenics' – special exercises to give good posture, usually taught by a man. Miss Buss (founder of the Girls Public Day School Trust) thought that callisthenics were very suitable for females:

. . . easy, graceful and not too fatiguing, gently calling every part of the body into play, by bright spirited music which cultivates rhythm of movement. (*Frances Mary Buss* by Annie Ridley, 1895, quoted in *Women First*)

Madame Osterberg, who was trained in Sweden, had introduced the Ling method of gymnastics for women into Britain by the end of the nineteenth century. She believed it was important to wear special clothes for exercising, and her first pupils wore 'blue serge tunics and knickerbockers, with light blue sashes round their waists' (*Daily News*, July 1884). The tunics were designed by a pupil, Mary Tait. Although

important physical fitness was for women.

> . . . Women are not healthy . . . . . it is a rare thing to meet with a lady of any age who does not suffer from headaches, languor, hysteria, or some ailment showing a want of stamina. (*On Secondary Instruction as Relating to Girls 1864*, quoted in *Sport and the Physical Emancipation of English Women*)

Students at Girton were encouraged to take part in gymastics, to swim, walk and play tennis, rackets, fives, croquet and badminton. Hockey was not introduced until 1890 and golf, cricket and lacrosse followed. A similar pattern developed at other universities and public schools, and by the end of the nineteenth century, games-playing and matches took place in schools for boys and girls alike. The pioneers of female education emphasized that games would improve a girl's health and child-bearing potential and would also instil in her valuable moral qualities.

Cycling was another activity which did much to promote women's liberation and was one of the first forms of physical activity which the middle classes in particular took up with enthusiasm. Female pioneer cyclists had to put up with a good deal of disapproval and were regularly ridiculed by the press and by *Punch* magazine in particular.

23 Girls take part in the fund-raising 'I Ran the World' contest, 1980s. Marathon running for women was only accepted as an Olympic sport in 1984.

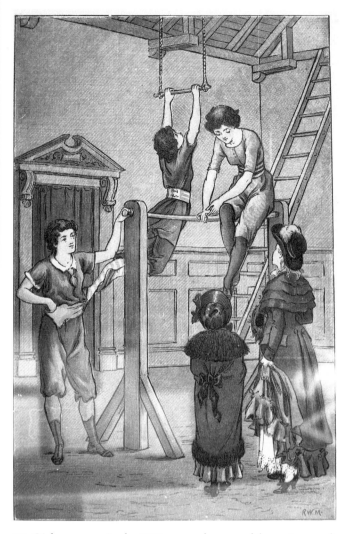

22 Girl gymnasts in the 1880s wear the type of dress pioneered by Madam Osterberg.

at first used strictly in private, the 'gym slip' became the accepted uniform for schoolgirls between the two world wars. One of the most important ways sport has helped to improve women's health has been the liberating influence it has had on their clothing.

Madame Osterberg, who had great drive and enthusiasm, publicized the Ling system by giving public gymnastic displays, and her teachers went into girls' board schools, public schools and universities. In 1885 she opened the Hampstead Physical Training College and Gymnasium, and ten years later the college moved to Dartford Heath.

Girls in the public schools and universities were also becoming interested in sports, which many had first learnt from their brothers during the holidays. Emily Davies, founder of Girton College, Cambridge, was one of the first educational pioneers to realize how

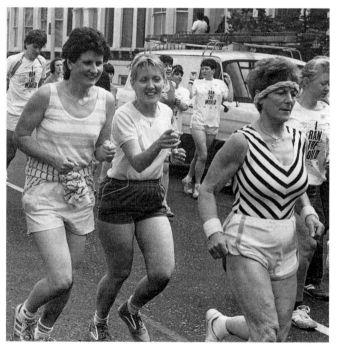

When lovely woman stoops to wheeling
And finds too late that bikes betray,
Beauty, grace and finer feeling
She'll see her sex has chucked away.
(*Punch*, 1890s, quoted in *Sport and the Physical Emancipation of English Women*)

Madame Osterberg included sports as well as gymnastics in her training programme at Dartford – athletics, cycling, tennis, lacrosse, netball and cricket were all on the curriculum. By the time she died in 1915, the College had become the leading physical education college for teachers, and her system was being taught all over Britain. Among the other female colleges, whose methods varied, were the Chelsea College of Physical Training, funded by Dorette Wilke, and the Anstey College of Physical Training and Hygiene for Women Teachers, founded in 1897 by Rhoda Anstey, one of Madame Osterberg's old pupils.

The College which was to have the most influence on future developments in the field of women's physical education was Bedford Physical Training College, founded by another of Osterberg's graduates, Margaret Stansfeld, in 1903. Ms Stansfeld's discipline was strict. Pupils were taught anatomy, physiology, hygiene, gymnastics, teaching methods, sport and games. She also founded the Ling Association, which dealt with salaries as well as training, and was its president from 1910 to 1920.

The Ling method, which dominated the years when women first began to take physical training, was developed entirely by women and with women in mind. It provided new job opportunities but it also isolated women within a rigid sexist system of training for a good many years.

There was a reaction against the Ling system between the wars, and even at Bedford College there were demands for less rigid methods and the inclusion of music in exercises. At the same time, a popular movement in favour of women's fitness grew up, and adult women of all social classes joined Keep Fit and the Women's League of Health and Beauty. The physical training colleges at first looked down on these new recruits to exercise, but later Miss Stansfeld suggested that some of her staff from Bedford College could help with the classes.

In the 1950s the Laban methods of training, which were closely connected with the modern dance movement, superceded Ling. Joan Goodrich, who succeeded Miss Stansfeld at Bedford College shortly before the war, was an enthusiastic supporter of the method. After the war all physical training colleges were assimilated into the educational system and started providing degree courses.

The history of women in athletics followed a similar pattern to that set in other sports. The founder of the modern Olympic Games, Baron Pierre de Coubertin, opposed the entry of women, who had to organize their own separate track and field events, the Women's

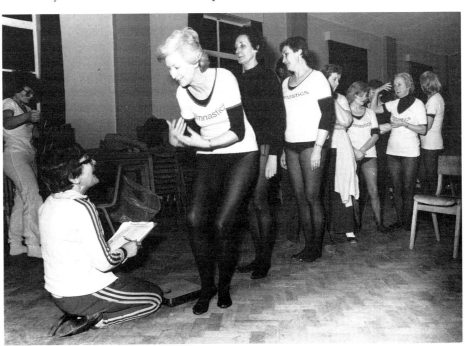

24 *Members of a Slimnastics class – a form of exercise started by Diana Lamplugh and Pamela Nottidge.*

World Games. It was only in 1928 that they were grudgingly allowed to compete, but following the collapse of Lina Radke after breaking the 800 metre world record for women, all women's track events, except for the 100 metres, were banned. The 200 metres was only reinstated in 1948, the 400 in 1964, the 800 in 1960 and the 1500 in 1972. The marathon and the 3000 were only included in 1984.

Most women did not often play games or take much exercise after leaving school until recently, when the new interest in physical fitness has made exercise into

a thriving industry. There are now increased facilities for playing squash and tennis and there are exercise classes using a wide variety of different techniques, for example Jane Fonda's aerobics, Diana Lamplugh's Slimnastics and Callan Pinckney's Callanetics. Jogging, marathon running and weight training have been taken up by men and women of all ages. Clothes have also become sports-orientated and tracksuits, leotards and trainers are now high-fashion garments. It is difficult to imagine today the inactive life lived by most women in the Victorian period.

Evidence

A (i) The bicycle is the greatest emancipator for women extant – women who long to be free from nervousness, headaches and all the trial of other ills. The wheel stimulates the circulation and regulates the action of the digestive canal, thus driving away headaches, and as a cure for nervousness it stands unrivalled. In every motion which the rider makes, the muscles are brought into play and gently exercised. With head and shoulders erect, those of the chest and arms are given a chance, while the pedal motion gives ample play to those of the legs. (Female correspondent in *The Girls Own Paper*, August 1901)

(ii) I don't think any woman, unless an old maid, hankers after emancipation of that sort, which seems to mean that, mounted on her bike, a girl can ride away anywhere and do anything all alone, without either male friend or chaperone, that she can guide and protect herself and be as free and easy as the wind. Well, I can assert, without fear of contradiction, that no man can really and truly care for a girl of this independent character, nor for one who pretends she can do everything manly quite as well as a man, or more so. (Reply from Gordon Stables MD, RN, *The Girls Own Paper*, August 1901)

B So, if exercise is good for us, where do we start? We may feel quite content and well enough leading our sedentary, physically ideal lives, but we must not mislead ourselves – our bodies are made to move . . . When we were children, we could usually romp around naturally keeping our bodies supple,

using up our energy, getting warm and out of breath, testing our strength ability and stretch, practising our skill and agility, and occasionally releasing our tension through complete relaxation . . . As adults at work, we often lose this ability . . . Our bodies often reveal neglect and misuse . . . The internal muscles also suffer from lack of use . . . To ensure complete safety as well as maximum efficiency, exercises should use muscles and joints in the ways for which they were designed . . . (Diana Lamplugh, founder of the British Slimnastics Association)

C Women are being encouraged to take part in sporting activities . . . but the insidious cultural message that sport is for men (or surrogate men) has not diminished. Women are venturing into new areas, such as rugby, soccer, long-distance running, solo marathon sailing, weight lifting, horse racing and mountaineering. Paradoxically, at the same time as women who are successful in sport are challenging the traditional sporting ideas, they *still* have to face the misconception that sports de-feminise them, and cope with insinuations about their sexuality. Competitors dye their hair blonde, wear jewellery and sexy sportswear to collude in the femininity game . . . If a woman is successful at sport, her sex is questioned, and her muscular body, which is the instrument of her success, is viewed with disgust. (Jenny Thomas, *Spare Rib*, 15 February 1985)

Questions

1 Why did the writer of A(i) believe that the bicycle was a great emancipator for women?

2 Are any similar ideas expressed in A(ii) and C? Are they expressed from the same point of view? Is this surprising?

3 Why do you think that some sports are still regarded as exclusively male or female?

CHAPTER 6

Clothing

Gabrielle (Coco) Chanel (1883-1971)

Fashion does not exist unless it goes down into the streets. The fashion that remains in the salons has no more significance than a costume ball. (Gabrielle 'Coco' Chanel).

Gabrielle (nicknamed 'Coco') Chanel came from a poor family in the South of France. She entered the fashion business shortly before the First World War, opening a hat shop in Deauville with the help of an English friend, Boy Capel. Having had an unconventional upbringing on the fringes of the Music Hall as a young girl, she wanted above all to *look* respectable and felt ridiculous in the elaborate styles of the period.

Another friend, Etienne Balsan, was a horse-racing enthusiast and Chanel ordered herself copies of a man's hacking jacket and jodhpurs from a local tailor to go riding with him. The clothes were remarkable in an age when women wore the same fussy styles in summer and winter, for work or play.

Chanel's personal style, at first derived from men's tailored clothes, became distinctive and she was much admired by her male friends, whose ties and jackets she often borrowed. Her chance to design clothes for others as well as herself came in 1916 when she opened a salon in Paris.

Other women had also begun to rebel against the tyranny of fashion, which decreed long skirts made of heavy material, large hats, tight shoes with high heels, heavy underclothes and restrictive corsets. By the early twentieth century many women had jobs, took part in sport, rode bicycles and wanted more loosely fitting, shorter clothes which did not require corsets. It was even more important during the First World War for

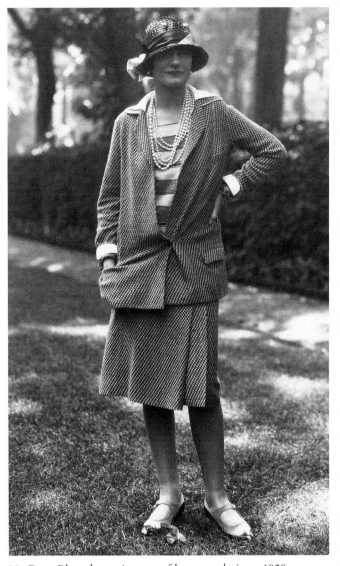

25 Coco Chanel wearing one of her own designs, 1929.

39

bus conductresses and others who had to move about quickly, to have garments that were not positively dangerous. Flowing dresses and long hair might catch in machinery with fatal results for female factory workers. Wartime uniforms also helped to do away with class distinctions in fashion.

Many of Chanel's designs were inspired by men's working clothing. They were at first known as the 'Poor Look'. She copied Breton sailors' sweaters, which were worn with simple jackets and pleated skirts. Silk squares tied at the neck echoed those worn by French stone masons. Mechanics' dungarees and sailors' bell-bottomed trousers were also adapted for women. Corsets were unnecessary for her easy-fitting styles.

Women were also beginning to wear their hair shorter, which went well with Chanel's clothes. The materials used were light – the weight of Edwardian clothes must have made even a brisk walk exhausting. Chanel used machine-made jersey, bought in bulk from a manufacturer who was trying to get rid of it – he had at first hoped to use the material for underclothes.

Chanel's style was essentially young and classless, looking best in the fresh air. In 1926 the American *Vogue* described one of her dresses as 'The Chanel "Ford" – the frock that all the world will wear'. She helped to create a market for leisure wear, which had not existed before the First World War. People had worn basically the same clothes for all occasions, including the beach, and even children were covered up from head to foot at all times.

Another advantage of Chanel's styles was that their simplicity made them adaptable for the mass market, and home dressmakers could copy the look using simple patterns. She made cardigans and sweaters fashionable. Lighter materials and separates were easy to wash. Pre-war garments had often smelt as they could only be dry-cleaned from time to time.

Chanel's clothes never really went out of fashion, although her influence declined in the later 1930s and during the Second World War. There was a major revival of her fortunes in 1954, for reasons similar to those which had first made her popular in the 1920s. Once more fashion had become middle-aged, expensive and formal. Julia Pascal remembered the restrictive clothes she had to wear when she was nine during the 1950s:

> My mother puts a roll-on [an elasticated corset] on my bed – 'to hold you in'. She wears one and I hate it but, because she tells me, I wear it. (*Truth, Dare or Promise*, edited by Liz Heron)

Chanel's designs liberated women a second time and copies were comparatively cheap to buy in Britain as they were retailed by the Wallis chain.

Although Gabrielle Chanel died in 1971, her salon continues under the direction of Karl Lagerfeld. As in Gabrielle's day, a whole range of products are marketed under the label, including handbags, shoes, jewellery and perfume.

> She is already influencing everything. At seventy-one Gabrielle Chanel is creating more than a fashion: a revolution. (*Life*, 1954)

Questions

1 In what ways were the Chanel's designs revolutionary? How were they beneficial to women's health?
2 In your opinion, did women's fashions since Chanel's time continue to be practical? Are they today?

Fashion and Health

Women's health and liberation are closely connected with fashion. The more elaborate a woman's clothes, the less she is able to do physically. In the Victorian period, fashion played on the myth of women's fragility and their supposed need of male protection – this reduced their credibility when women began to compete with men in the professions and in business.

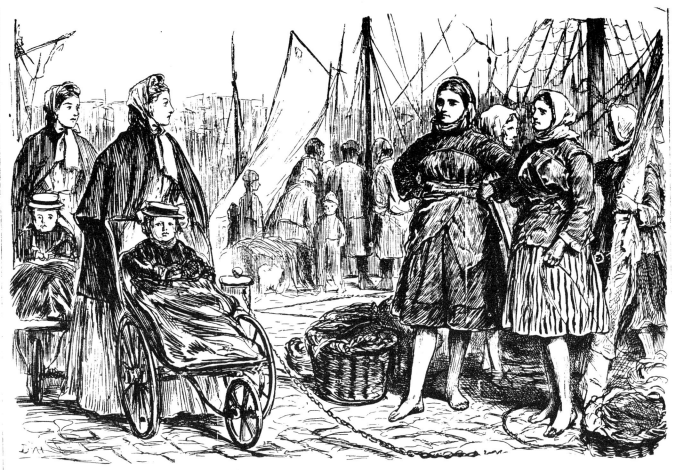

" HONI SOIT," &c.

ANN AND SARAH SEE SOME FISHWOMEN "CLOTHED *THAT* INDELICATE THAT YOU MIGHT HAVE KNOCKED THEM DOWN WITH A FEATHER!"

Working-class women were not usually concerned with fashion in the nineteenth century. They seldom wore corsets, except sometimes for best. It was not until wages improved, mass-produced clothes were available and materials became cheaper that there was any money to spare for fashion. Working clothes such as those worn by Victorian fishergirls, women miners or farm labourers, were strictly practical. Women coal pit workers in Wigan, for instance, were wearing trousers in the mid-nineteenth century, according to evidence given to the Select committee on Mines in 1866. In 1886 a local vicar expressed the opinion that:

. . . In twenty years time they would be looked up on as the pioneers of civilisation in the matter of women's dress . . . he admired their courage in wearing it, and wished there was equal courage to be found in women at the top of the social scale. (Quoted in Michael Hiley's *Victorian Working Women*, Gordon Fraser Gallery, 1979).

26 While middle-class women were tightly corseted and wore long skirts in 1866, the Boulogne fisher girls wore less constricting garments.

Dress has a disproportionate amount of influence on the social assessment of men and women. Fashionable women's clothes were generally designed with two purposes in mind – to show off the wealth of the family or to attract the opposite sex. Dress can also have political or religious implications. Victorian women's clothes spelt out female subjugation and class distinction. The fashion industry was also based on the exploitation of women in the garment and textile factories. Friedrich Engels described in the 1840s:

[Women] who sleep and eat on the premises, come usually from the country and are therefore absolutely the slaves of their employers. (*The Condition of the Working Class in England*, 1844)

41

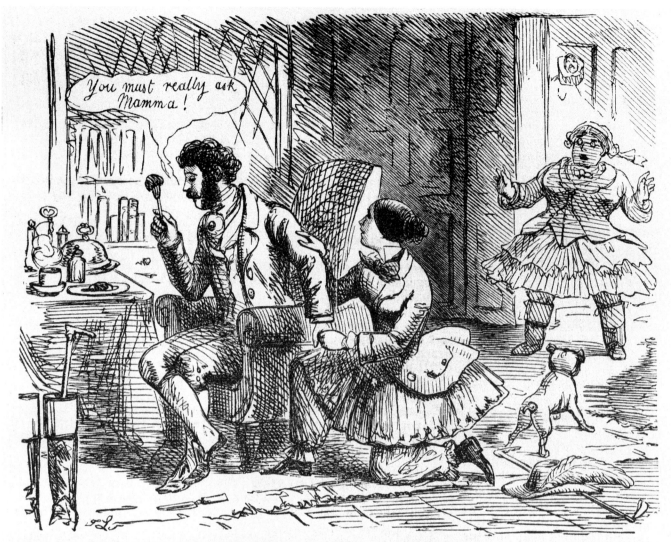

ONE OF THE DELIGHTFUL RESULTS OF BLOOMERISM.—THE LADIES WILL POP THE QUESTION.

27 A Punch *cartoon of the 1850s illustrates what men feared might happen if women wore the trousers.*

By the early nineteenth century women were wearing a heavy assortment of garments including several petticoats, often made of flannel, a wheel of horsehair to make the skirt stand out (later replaced by a hoop) and stays, which were tightly laced. Women could not move their bodies much – in fact it was said of one girl, who tried to pick something up from the floor:

Her stays gave way with a tremendous explosion, and she fell to the ground. I thought she had snapped in two. (Quoted in *The Bloomer Girls*)

As a result of tight lacing and not much fresh air, women frequently fainted and had an 'interesting pallor' which was much admired. A woman's place was in the home and she dressed to show that she was incapable of travelling far outside it.

From the early nineteenth century, some medical men had campaigned against the unhealthy and unhygienic aspects of women's clothes.

No woman who dresses tightly can have good shoulders, a straight spine, good lungs, sweet breath, and be perfectly healthy. (Written by a critic of tight lacing in a ladies' magazine, quoted in *The Bloomer Girls*)

Amelia Bloomer (1818-1894) was an American pioneer who fought for less restricting clothes in the 1850s, as she thought that current fashions were symbolic of female repression. Her remedy was a shorter skirt worn with trousers 'cut moderately full and gathered in above the footwear'. 'Bloomers' were immediately denounced as immoral and there is no doubt that men found the idea of women wearing trousers threatening. Ms Bloomer had become a member of the Women's Rights Movement in America in 1850, editing their journal, *The Lily*. One early article in the journal was by Elizabeth Cády Stanton, who wrote:

> What use is all the flummery, puffing, and mysterious folding we see in ladies' dress? . . . If women for the last fifty years had spent all the time they have wasted on furbelowing their rags, in riding, walking, and playing on the lawn with their children, the whole race would look ten times as well as they now do!

Ms Bloomer based her ideas of dress on a costume designed by a friend to wear travelling in Switzerland, which included loose Turkish trousers and a short skirt. Ms Stanton described her feelings after trying out the garments for the first time in America:

> Like a captive set free from his ball and chain, I was always ready for a brisk walk through sleet and snow and rain, to climb a mountain, jump over a fence, work in the garden . . . What a sense of liberty I felt . . . (Quoted in *The Bloomer Girls*)

Ms Bloomer wore the costume herself and announced it to readers of *The Lily*. Her article received a lot of female support and her ideas reached Britain in 1851. Bloomers were ridiculed mercilessly in the press and music-halls and soon died a natural death. The American pioneers also gave up the struggle because they felt that too much publicity about dress had taken attention away from the true goals of female emancipation: the need for better education; better job opportunities; equal pay; and the right to vote.

By the 1880s, sport was beginning to influence both male and female fashion, and bloomers were revived as they were particularly suitable for women cycling enthusiasts. Female explorers like Mary Kingsley and Isabella Bird had often enterprisingly designed their own costumes, which had to be sufficiently modest to be accepted by primitive communities but also practical for climbing over gates and up mountains. Fashion was also now being influenced by women who were entering the professions or working in offices and therefore favoured tailored clothes.

In spite of women's widening horizons, fashion did not become progressively more liberated, as from time to time women deliberately put themselves back into awkward, restricting garments. Tennis player Betty Ryan remembers how some women were still wearing steel-boned corsets at tennis tournaments just before the First World War. 'It was never a pretty sight, for most of them were bloodstained' (quoted in Teddy Tinling, *60 Years in Tennis*).

Although women's clothes became healthier and more comfortable during the 1920s, Dior's 'New Look', after the Second World War, brought back corseted, impractical, ultra-feminine styles, which were welcomed by women themselves as a contrast to

28 Women's Liberation campaigners protest against the symbols of female subjugation, which include items of dress.

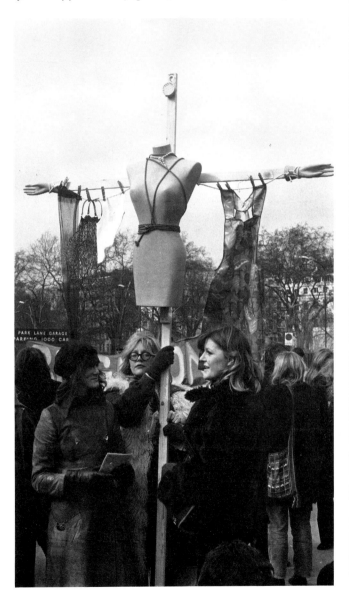

wartime austerity. Gwen Hughes, a Lancashire mill girl at the time, remembered:

> I had a navy blue coat, nipped in at the waist and ankle length with a very full skirt. With it I wore strap-round-the-ankle lizard-skin, wedge-heeled shoes and huge fur-backed gloves. Of course, I always wore a hat, that goes without saying. (Quoted in *Out of the Doll's House*)

In the 1980s fashions became more varied. Even the corsets, stockings, and suspenders thankfully discarded by women of the 1960s have returned to a certain extent. At the same time, there has been a trend towards more comfortable casual fashions inspired by the modern passion for health and sport. The real revolution which has taken place is that fashion is no longer followed slavishly, and is now more a matter of personal choice.

A ruff in the Elizabethan period and a fur coat in the 1930s were both status symbols, and women are still judged by the clothes they wear.

Evidence

A **Balloons of the Ball** Ladies' dresses are generally airy at this time of year, but those of the present season are particularly so . . . A gentleman . . . describes himself as having attended at the late Imperial baptismal ball at the Hôtel de Ville. The immense circumference of the skirts thereat exhibited, astounded him; and by his account it appears that the expansion of female drapery has become so excessive as to constitute the wearer a perfect nuisance to herself . . . It renders the exertion of getting into and out of a carriage a difficulty amounting to perfect trial, and its inconvenience is bitterly complained of by many of the sufferers whom an imperious necessity compels to submit thereto. (*Punch*, 5 July 1856)

B She had been brought up in service, she said; but of her own accord had left that calling, and gone down a coal pit, about 15 years ago, to work as a drawer . . . Of course she went as a man; dressed in men's clothes and passed as a man . . . All this the handsome brighteyed woman told with quiet unaffected candour. 'I liked it!' she said with emphasis: 'but when I'd been working down a month, they found out I was a woman, and I was turned out; and since then I've worked on pit-brow and worn breeches as I'm doing now'.

She laughed at her grotesque attire: 'such queer old clothes as we wear!' said she 'ragged ones that folks gie us – our brothers' old coats and breeches – anything does to work at pit in; but we wear our breeches always, yo know, 'cept Sundays – and nice and warm, they are too'. (Arthur Munby's diary, 19 August 1963, quoted in Michael Hiley's *Victorian Working Women*, 1979)

C During the war the women took the men's role. They worked in factories and they ran the home. Then after the war, they wanted to go back to being pretty, feminine 'little women' again, and being looked after by the men. And perhaps this was sort of encouraged because when the men came back from the war, they wanted their jobs back, so the women had to be sort of pushed back into the home, didn't they? (Woman who was a teenager during the Second World War, quoted in *You'll Never Be 16 Again*)

Questions

1 How do the clothes of the women described in A and B reflect their social class and society's expectations of them?

2 With refence to C, explain why women chose to go back to wearing 'feminine' clothes after the Second World War? Why is it that women are often still judged by the clothes they wear?

3 Can you think of any situations in which a certain type of dress is demanded? Are these clothes always practical?

CHAPTER 7

Stress

Diana Lamplugh (b. 1936)

Health is affected by one's state of mind as well as by physical factors. Many of these mental and psychological problems are today grouped together under the word 'stress'. Some medical conditions like heart trouble or stomach ulcers, which seem to people untrained in medicine to be purely physical, are now described as 'stress-related diseases'. People turn to drugs, alcohol or smoking because of too much stress. In the past, men in high-pressure jobs were the most likely sufferers, but now women are catching up. Women may also have the additional stress of sexual harrassment at work and the danger of violence in the street.

Stress takes many forms. In Diana Lamplugh's case, her crusade to protect woman from violence directed against them at work was a consequence of her daughter Suzy's disappearance – a 25-year-old estate agent who vanished after an appointment with a client in 1986. When Ms Lamplugh founded the Suzy Lamplugh Trust, she felt she was making a positive response and that good might come out of evil if she prevented other women from suffering the same fate as her daughter. Her own grief and stress when Suzy disappeared were partly alleviated by her activities for the Trust.

Diana Lamplugh worked as a secretary before her marriage, and Suzy, who was born in 1961, was the second of her four children. Her husband Paul was a solicitor and the family lived in Sheen, Surrey. When her children were young, Ms Lamplugh qualified as a swimming instructor and in 1973 she and Pamela Nottidge founded the British Slimnastics Association, which advocated a holistic (whole person) approach to physical fitness through exercises, diet, relaxation and tension control. Groups were set up all over the country and today the BSA has 300 Slimnastics Teachers and a grant from the Sports Council. Ms Lamplugh continues to act as Consultant and Assessor. Slimnastics, like other exercise systems, does much to alleviate stress and provides guidance in other aspects of general health.

When her daughter failed to come back from a lunch-time appointment with a client, Diana Lamplugh and her family suddenly became front-page news in the national press. The disappearance also revealed the potential dangers for women in that kind

29 Diana Lamplugh, who founded the Suzy Lamplugh Trust in 1986, primarily to protect women at work from sexual aggression and harassment.

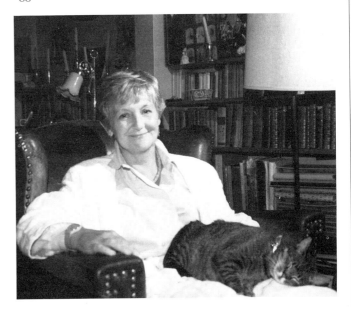

of work. Early on in the investigations Ms Lamplugh decided that it was no use keeping a low profile. She felt that the only way to get a result was to keep the case firmly in the public eye and she was adept at dealing with the media. A few months after Suzy's disappearance she founded the Suzy Lamplugh Trust, converting the top floor of her house into an office. Diana Lamplugh defined the need for such an organization:

> When Suzy made that routine call on a Monday lunchtime in July last year, purely acting in her role as negotiator, it seems she was off guard and did not sense her vulnerability . . . (reported in Andrew Stephen, *The Suzy Lamplugh Story*)

The Trust's aims are to to protect women at work from sexual aggression and harassment, to make women more generally aware of the danger of violence inside and outside the home and to help the relatives of missing persons. Towards this end the Trust provides training schemes, videos, books, personal alarms, educational packs and courses on role play, assertiveness and male-female working relationships. In theory its policies are applicable to both men and women. Ms Lamplugh now lectures all over the country, broadcasts on radio and television and arranges fundraising events. She has also started a campaign to have mini-cabs registered.

A report by the London School of Economics, *The Risks in Going to Work*, was funded by the Trust and published in March 1989. It stresses the need for classes to raise women's awareness about potential dangers and recommends that in the case of occupations such as Suzy's, when a woman is more at risk than a man, that a companion should be taken to appointments. The report also suggests that all appointments should be clearly logged and that there should be a recognized follow-up procedure if the worker does not come back at the expected time. The conclusions are that many women suffer stresses of various kinds at work and that there is a high level of anxiety in the younger age group.

Sexual harassment emerges as a problem for women. The proportion of women likely to encounter sexual harassment in the course of their work is one in seven . . . but, for women in professional occupations which involve a substantial amount of time away from the office, and those working in shops and offices, the proportion is one in five . . . The majority of women who experienced sexual harassment were angry; many felt depressed and less efficient at work; and some did not want to go to work or developed physical symptoms of stress. (Dr C.M. Phillips, Dr J.E. Stockdale, *The Risks in Going to Work*).

To date the mystery of Suzy Lamplugh's disappearance has not been solved. Diana Lamplugh continues her work for the Trust, has written a number of books, including *Slimnastics* (with Pamela Nottidge), *Stress and Overstress* (1974), *Beating Aggression* (1988) and *Survive the 9-5* (1989). She has recently completed a video, *Avoiding Danger*. She believes that the work of the Trust is a logical progression from her slimnastics philosophy: 'Without health, strength and the ability to relax, you are not able to look after yourself'.

Diana Lamplugh's own answer to the grief and stress caused by the disappearance of her daughter was to launch the Trust. One of the worst aspects of the story is that the family may never know what happened to Suzy. Diana's self-control broke when Andrew Stephen's book about the case (*The Suzy Lamplugh Story*) was written in 1988, and the Lamplughs tried to stop publication. Diana Lamplugh has described her 'double bereavement' – the actual loss of her daughter and the emotional loss because of the book. She felt that the author gave a misleading view of her daughter's emotional life, and cast doubts on her own reasons for launching the Trust and encouraging publicity through the media.

Diana Lamplugh has had to go back painfully over her motives. She admits that she enjoyed the media attention but felt it was a way of taking the only positive action open to her and the opportunity to prevent other women from suffering the same tragedy as her daughter.

Questions

1 What methods did Diana Lamplugh use to combat her own stress?

2 How can sport and exercise help to beat stress?

3 Why do the courses Diana Lamplugh runs cover aspects such as assertiveness and male-female working relationships? Why are women vulnerable to sexual harassment?

Pressures at Home and Work

Stress is a word often used today but it does not necessarily describe a disease of the modern world. It is only the type of stress that has sometimes changed. The stresses suffered by women have often been the result of their position in society, and society's expectations of them. Before it was acceptable for middle-class women to go out to work, far more suffered from 'nerves' and depression. Dorothea Beale wrote in the late nineteenth century:

> I am quite certain that there would be less illness amongst the upper classes if their brains were more regularly and systematically worked. (Quoted in *Out of the Doll's House*)

Before the Women's Liberation Movement gained momentum in the 1960s, few married women were given much sympathy for nervous problems or tiredness and depression. Betty Friedan believes that after the Second World women were expected to fit in to a masculine dream image of a housewife who found her fulfilment in the home. A job was not part of the picture, and increasing numbers suffered from both psychological and physiological problems. Betty Friedan quotes some of the symptoms:

> A tired feeling . . . I get so angry with the children it scares me . . . I feel like crying without any reason. (A Cleveland doctor called it 'the housewife's syndrome') A number of women told me about great bleeding blisters that break out on their hands and arms. 'I call it the housewife's blight', said a family doctor in Pennsylvania. 'I see it so often lately in these young women with four, five and six children who bury themselves in their dishpans. But it isn't caused by detergent and it isn't cured by cortisone'. (*The Feminine Mystique*).

30 The 'tonic wine' Wincarnis was often taken to relieve the stresses of being a housewife in the twenties and thirties.

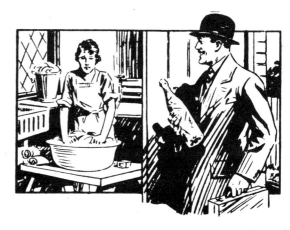
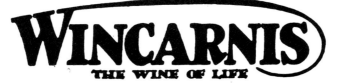

Women often had nobody to turn to to seek help for such seemingly inexplicable complaints. Before modern support and self-help groups were set up, many women used the only advice service available to them – the 'problem pages' in women's magazines. 'Agony aunts' would attempt to sort out emotional and stress-related problems expressed in readers' distraught letters with one short reply.

The doctors' answer to the so-called 'housewife's syndrome' in the 1950s was to give their patients pills. There have always been medicines reputed to cure nervous and emotional problems. In the Victorian period most of them contained opium. Some of the drugs prescribed in post-war Britain were equally addictive, although not recognized as such at the time. Tranquillizers such as Valium and Ativan were widely prescribed for depression or sleeplessness. There are still horrific stories about women who have been prescribed tranquillizers for the past twenty years and are now totally dependent on them.

Professor Ian Stanley of Liverpool University discovered from his research that more women than men were prescribed drugs, usually for a '. . . period of life crisis. Typically in an older woman during, or after, a bereavement and they'd just never been stopped. Patients, I think, didn't realise that they were dependent on them . . .' (quoted in *Out of the Doll's House*). Now self-help groups like TRANX, started by Anita Gordon, an ex victim of Valium, are helping

31 Notices on the door of a women's refuge reflect the terrible pressures faced by women with violent husbands.

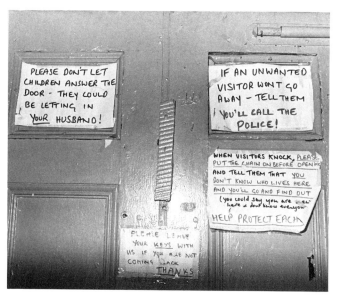

these women to give up the pills and return to normal life.

> The drugs ensure that the anxiety remains, so that it all surges back up again when you stop taking them. I was going through very severe withdrawal symptoms. Part of the problem was that, while on the drugs I did feel confident and able to cope, yet I was only half alive. (Anita Gordon, quoted in Liz Hodgkinson, *Addictions*)

The addictive problems of alcohol, smoking and hard drugs are suffered by men and women alike and there are many different forms of treatment. More girls now smoke than boys, with the result that lung cancer in women has increased. DAWN (Drugs, Alcohol, Women, Nationally), a charity which helps women to deal with addictive problems, says in its leaflet *Women and Heroin*:

> Women start to use heroin for a lot of different reasons. It cushions us from reality, makes problems fade away and at first can give us confidence and energy. Many women use it in the long term to get through routine tasks, such as housework, coping with a family or a boring job, or to cope with an otherwise intolerable situation.

The general increase in addictive habits and stress-related diseases among women is thought to be related to the increased number of women in top jobs, many of whom are still largely responsible for running the home and bringing up the family.

Although both men and women suffer from stress-related diseases, there are some stresses which are considered to be particular to women. Diana Lamplugh and Erin Pizzey have drawn attention to sex-related violence in the home and workplace. Erin Pizzey was one of the first to understand that women with violent husbands needed counselling and a place to stay with their children. She opened Chiswick Women's Aid in 1971, which became known popularly as the Battered Wives Centre. Today the organization she started is known as Chiswick Family Rescue, and since 1983 has been directed by Sandra Horley.

Another group dealing with related problems is the feminist Women Against Violence Against Women, which was set up in 1980 after the Yorkshire Ripper murders, to protest against pornography and its connection with violence. The Rape Crisis Centre, Women Against Rape and Women Against Sexual Harrassment have also been formed. Feminists like Sheila Jeffreys believes that sexual violence has increased in proportion to women's liberation and is used as a weapon to 'keep women in their place'.

Stress would not occur if everyone was perfectly content all the time. The make-up artist Barbar Daly believes that people should practise the art of 'stress management' and use whatever method they think best – exercise, hobbies, an encounter group, meditation or alternative medicine.

> I meditate for up to an hour every morning . . . I practise Siddha meditation which . . . slows down the pulse rate and breathing and makes me feel very much more centred . . . I sleep better and my asthma has improved. I used to suffer from a nervous stomach and indigestion but that's gone too . . . (Barbara Daly, interviewed in the *Guardian*, 16 February 1990).

Evidence

A Keeping faith

'Please help me, you can't imagine my trouble. My boy has been a prisoner in Japan for three years and I can't go out with other boys when I think of what he may be suffering. All my girl friends are courting now and I am so lonely I don't know what to do.'

Poor little girl, it is terrible that this, which should be your happiest time, should be so clouded. But I am glad that you are keeping faith with your boy . . . Isn't there a youth club you could join and make new friends? Or how about volunteering at any local canteen several nights a week? (War-time issue of *Woman's Own*, 7 July 1944)

B Of course the main difference between male and female managers is that for most women their working day does not end at 5.00 pm. How many men spend their lunch times queuing in the supermarket or dashing round to collect the dry-cleaning? Running even a two-person household takes more time and energy than is generally realized and it is not uncommon for me to spend four or five hours a day on matters connected with a home . . . For women with young families the demands on their energy and patience must be enormous and we should hardly be surprised if they do complain of fatigue and feel torn between the demands of home and work. Hilary, Manager in charge of a Job Centre since 1981, quoted in *Stress and the Woman Manager* by Marilyn Davidson and Cary Cooper).

C I was getting pretty crazy and nobody really noticed . . . But the way doctors are trained, they find it very difficult to ask for help. My father came to talk to the consultant who said he thought I'd been a bit off, but he assumed it was boyfriend trouble. A lot of the difficulties were in me, but they weren't helped by being in a stressful, irregular sort of job and I felt very lost in London . . . I found that [drink] relieved anxiety and tension and gave me confidence. (Woman doctor, quoted in the *Guardian*, 9 February 1990).

D Tranquillisers, I came to learn, blunt the whole of your perception . . . The drugs ensure that the anxiety remains, so that it all surges back up again when you stop taking them. Part of the problem was that, while on the drugs I did feel confident and able to cope, yet I was only half alive. When I go out into the garden now I am aware of things growing, but I simply didn't notice them before. I feel now that those fifteen years were wasted, spent as a zombie and not really living at all . . . I don't actually think that emotional difficulties, such as I was going through, can be treated medically. Personal help and advice is the answer. (Anita Gordon, who was prescribed Valium for fifteen years, and who has now started Tranks, to help others with similar problems; quoted in *Addictions* by Liz Hodgkinson, Thorsons Publishing Group, 1986).

Questions

1 How helpful is the advice of magazine 'agony aunts' such as that of source A?

2 What causes of stress at work are expressed in B and C? Why are women so often torn between the demands of home and work?

3 Why were tranquillizers prescribed as a cure for stress? Do you think we have a better understanding of (a) the causes and (b) the appropriate treatment of stress today?

4 Do you agree that women are more likely to suffer from stress than men?

CHAPTER 8

Childbirth

Wendy Savage (b. 1935)

Pregnancy is not an illness. I belong to the school of thought which believes that every pregnancy is normal unless there are indications that something is wrong. Those at the opposite end of the obstetric spectrum believe that no pregnancy is normal, except in retrospect. (Wendy Savage, *A Savage Enquiry*)

Wendy Savage was trained at Girton College, Cambridge, and the London Hospital. She married shortly after taking her final exams, moving to the USA in 1962 where she worked as a research assistant at the Boston City Hospital. When her husband's job took her and their three children to Nigeria, she studied obstetrics and gynaecology and decided to specialize. Leaving Nigeria when the Biafran war broke out, Dr Savage worked in Kenya for a short while before returning to England and becoming a member of the Royal College of Obstetricians and Gynaecologists in 1969.

For the next seven years Wendy Savage worked in areas which she felt had been neglected in orthodox training, such as family planning, sterilization, abortion and venereal disease. She was also with the Pregnancy Advisory Service for a year. Between 1973 and 1976 she practised in New Zealand. She became a lecturer at the London Hospital Medical College in 1976 and in 1977 was appointed Senior Lecturer and Honorary Consultant in Obstetrics and Gynaecology at the London Hospital. In April 1985 she was suspended from her clinical work, pending an enquiry into her competence.

The background to Wendy Savage's suspension was a difference in attitudes towards the treatment of women in labour, which had divided the medical

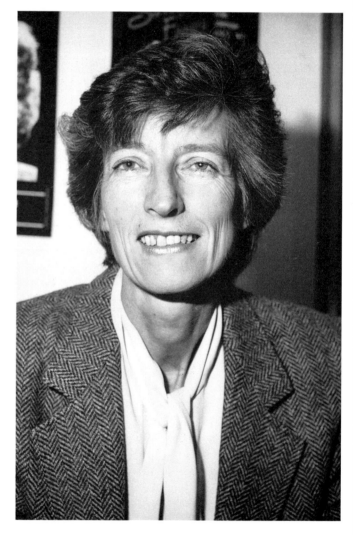

32 Dr Wendy Savage shortly after she was reinstated as consultant Obstetrician and Gynaecologist at the London Hospital in 1989.

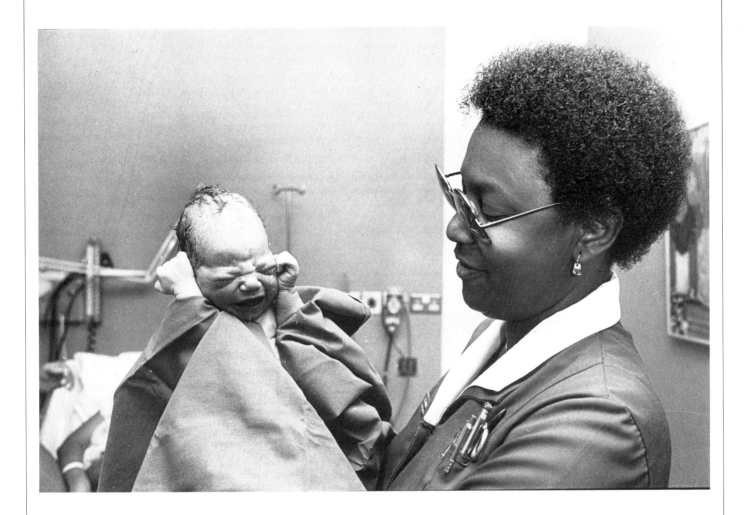

33 A hospital midwife with a new-born baby. Most births in Britain today take place in a hospital and not at home.

world and women themselves since the 1960s. With the improvements in surgical techniques and the development of new drugs, childbirth had become much safer, but control had passed from the home-based, female midwife to the generally male clinician working in hospital.

Wendy Savage believed that women should have the opportunity to feel in control of the birth process and should not be forced into, say, having a baby by surgery (Caesarean section), unless in an emergency. Working in Professor Peter Huntingford's unit at the London Hospital, Dr Savage had tried to offer women a choice of services by sharing antenatal care with GPs and by encouraging midwives to take on home deliveries. She had also helped to provide a day-care abortion service, which had aroused some opposition. After Professor Huntingford moved to Maidstone in 1981, in-fighting in the Department of Obstetrics and Gynaecology left Wendy Savage outnumbered by those who opposed her methods.

Reading the suspension papers, Wendy Savage found:

> . . . my management of labour is said to give rise to serious concern about the safety of patients in my care. I think: this isn't about competence, it's about attitudes, about a different approach to maternity care. (*A Savage Enquiry*)

After her immediate suspension on April 24 1985, Wendy Savage prepared for the public enquiry, which was held in February 1986. Her case received wide press coverage and a Wendy Savage Support Group was formed which included many of her former patients. Beverley Beech and Sheila Kitzinger of the National Childbirth Trust gave their support and added to the media coverage. An Appeal Fund Committee was formed to raise money for legal fees.

Five specific cases were cited by the opposition. In four of them a Caesarean section had only been undertaken after labour had been tried. Wendy Savage believed that surgery and induction (starting labour by surgical means) had been used too much in recent years. Apart from the dangers inherent in any surgery, these mothers were more prone to depression after birth and had difficulty in relating to their babies. Above all, she felt that: 'Women are different, and each woman and each labour should be managed individually'.

The trial lasted 25 days and the report was not made public until 10 July 1986. Wendy Savage was completely cleared and on 24 July 1986 she was

reinstated. The debate about obstetric care continues and Wendy Savage believes obstetricians, midwives and ordinary women should join together in discussion to find 'how best to use resources and what women want'.

In 1989 Wendy Savage completed a report on women's attitudes and experiences in regard to cervical screening, her main recommendation being that a greater emphasis on the health aspects of the test should be made, rather than treating it primarily as a test for cancer. She also suggested the introduction of a women's health card.

Questions

1 Why did Wendy Savage's approach to her work 'give rise to serious concern'?

2 What problems arose when childbirth became more hospital orientated?

3 Why does Dr Savage believe it is important for a woman to have a choice in how she wants to have her baby?

Maternity Care

Historically, control of fertility and midwifery were in women's hands. Twentieth century medicine brought them under the aegis of doctors: an elitist, institutionally male profession. (Sally Hughes in the *Guardian*, August 1988)

Home-births, with a female midwife in attendance, were always the custom in the past and this is still predominantly the case in many parts of the Third World today. Methods of delivery and care have varied. Percivall Willughby noticed in 1863 that, 'Several midwives, chiefly about London, use midwives stools but elsewhere kneeling was the country mode of delivery' (quoted in Edward Shorter, *A History of Women's Bodies*). An upper-middle-class woman might have had one to two weeks in bed after giving birth but the working classes had only one or two days.

There was a high mortality rate among mothers and babies, who suffered from infection or birth complications. Willughby often found 'the mother undelivered, and she and the child dead before I could come unto them, through the ignorance of such

midwives'. The poor and unmarried could obtain treatment in 'lying-in' hospitals in the nineteenth century, where there was also a high mortality rate, often because puerperal fever spread from one mother to another in the wards.

A few men became midwives in the eighteenth century, but it was during the twentieth century that male doctors largely took over control of childbirth. Medicalization occurred because of scientific advances and because obstetrics and gynaeocology became recognized specialities when the British College of Obstetricians and Gynaeocologists was founded in 1929.

Although surgery helped to ease many of the more painful and dangerous conditions which can accompany childbirth, the number of Caesarian operations increased during the 1930s, some of which were no doubt unnecessary. General practitioners, who were now attending more births, had received little training in obstetrics and some had no idea how to carry out a forceps delivery. The Midwives Act (1936) created a professional, salaried midwifery service,

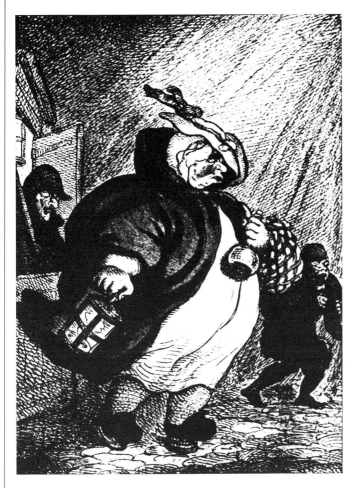

34 Rowlandson's caricature of a midwife going out on a case at the beginning of the nineteenth century.

administered by the local authorities, and midwives still retained control in some practices. The conditions under which they worked were often very bad. Beatrice Sandys, a trainee midwive during the period, remembers:

Whole families lived in one room . . . There was bugs and fleas and all that kind of thing. We were warned by the matron that when we went up the stairs we mustn't touch the walls with our clothes, we must walk in the middle of the stairs. (Quoted in *Out of the Doll's House*)

In spite of scientific advances, childbirth still had its dangers between the wars. W. Blair Bell, first president of the British College of Obstetricians and Gynaecologists, said in 1931 that at least ten per cent of all mothers suffered from disabling conditions as the result of childbirth.

Women began to press for improved maternal care. One of the pioneers, Janet Campbell (1877-1954),

became Senior Medical Officer to the Maternity and Child Welfare section of the Ministry of Health and in 1928 persuaded the Ministry to set up a Committee on Maternal Mortality and Morbidity, on which she served. The Committee's enquiries and those of the Women's Health Enquiry Committee – reported in Margery Spring Rice's book *Working Class Wives* (1939) – revealed that the poor standard of living among the working classes and unemployed prejudiced efficient antenatal care. Janet Campbell's books include *Maternal Mortality* (1924), *The Training of Midwives* (1923), *The Protection of Motherhood* (1927) and *Infant Mortality* (1929).

It's four times as dangerous to bear a child as to work in a mine; and mining is man's most dangerous trade. (Mary Stocks, speaking in the 1920s, quoted in *Out of the Doll's House*).

Living standards improved after the Second World War, and the establishment of the National Health Service in 1948 provided comprehensive antenatal, delivery and postnatal care. The first point of contact for a pregnant woman became her GP, not the midwife. Compared with 1937, when 40 per cent of British babies were born in hospital, in 1959 the figure had risen to 64 per cent, in 1972 to 91.4 per cent, and today only one per cent of babies are born at home. Midwives are now moving away from the community into hospital practice, although there are some independent midwives working outside the Health Service.

Medical intervention during labour has also increased since the last war. Although childbirth became safer, women wanted more control over their own bodies. Pressure groups were formed, among them the Natural Childbirth Trust, founded in Britain in 1956 to improve women's knowledge about childbirth and to help them deal with pain through special exercises. The Trust believes that a good birth is one achieved without drugs or obstetric intervention. Another pioneer was Suzann Arms in America, who believed that childbearing had been made unnatural in order to reduce risks (*Immaculate Deception* 1975). The social anthropologist Sheila Kitzinger has done much to form thinking about natural childbirth in Britain and has written a number of best-selling books about it and on female sexuality. In 1960 the Association for Improvements in the Maternity Services was founded by Sally Willmington to provide advice for women with problems associated with

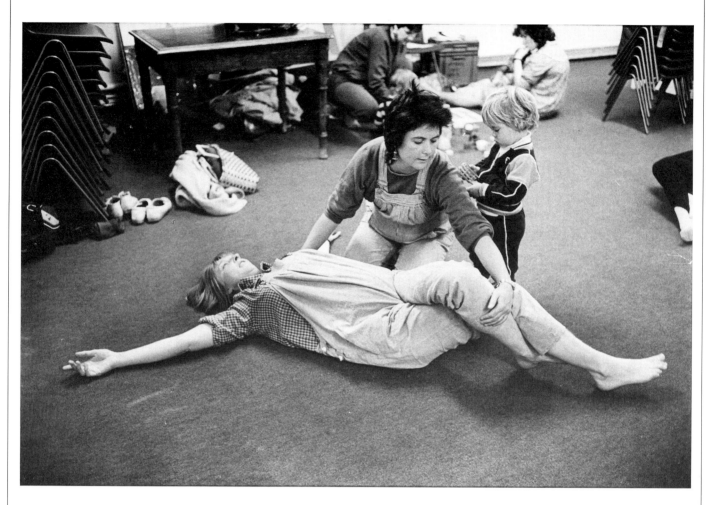

35 Women take part in an 'Active Birth' class, a popular method of preparing for childbirth today.

antenatal care. In the same year another pressure group, the Society for the Prevention of Cruelty to Pregnant Women (later called AIMS), was formed:

> We still receive reports from women of antenatal clinics described as cattle-markets . . . long sordid waits for a brief prod by a stranger (different each visit) who is hostile to women's questions about their own bodies. (AIMS Newsletter, 1980)

Midwives are under pressure today because of cuts in maternity services and poor pay. Several have made headlines recently because of their independent action. Jilly Rosser, who works for the Haringey Health Authority in North London, was suspended from the professional register for taking a haemorrhaging mother by car to hospital because she was afraid that the ambulance with an obstetric team would arrive too late. She was later reinstated after an inquiry. Caroline Flint, who acts as an independent midwife outside the

Health Service and consultant to Riverside Health Authority, has been reported to the midwives' investigating committee after dealing with an emergency in a home birth without a doctor being present.

> I believe all these cases . . . are about a conflict of philosophies over methods of childbirth. Hospitals have rigid procedures which are usually laid down by obstetricians, whereas independent midwives practise autonomously and in women's homes, providing all the necessary care from beginning to end. They are disproving the commonly held view that childbirth is a dangerous process requiring medical control. (Caroline Flint, quoted in the *Sunday Times*, July 1988).

There is, however, always the need to have a medical back-up to the midwife in case of complications requiring surgical procedures, which can only be carried out by an appropriately qualified doctor.

Some female obstetricians also have reservations about childbirth procedures. Apart from Wendy Savage, Pauline Bousquet, senior consultant obstetrician and gynaecologist for the City and Hackney Health Authority in London, was attacked for her policy of letting nature take its course when possible during labour. She was against induced labour or epidural analgesia (which anaesthetizes the back) as a matter of policy. Since the 1970s her obstetric and gynaecological sessions were whittled down and in 1987 she was made redundant.

The argument still continues, and in spite of the natural childbirth lobby, many women prefer to be in hospital and to have pain relief during labour, though some feel that they are failures, quite undeservedly, because they have been unable to follow the ideal of natural childbirth.

Evidence

A Witches were supposed to have special power over all that concerned fertility in man and nature . . . Midwives came under particular suspicion, probably because of their medical knowledge which, poor as it was in the Middle Ages and much later, was at least superior to that of their neighbours. They were generally accused, and probably with reason, of using spells to assist delivery . . . thirty years ago in one Somerset village a woman reputed to have the Evil Eye was preferred before the trained District Nurse at such times, partly because of her occult knowledge . . . Even in our own day, when the general belief in Witchcraft has almost died away, it is still said in parts of East Anglia that a midwife has some power which enables her always to arrive in time, no matter how far away she may be, and regardless of whether ordinary transport is available for her or not. (Christina Hole, writing in 1945, *Witchcraft in England*, Batsford)

B When I became a midwife there were no drugs. Some midwives gave them gin. The woman had a lot more pain then. You gave them a list of the things you needed – a big new saucepan to boil things up in and you took what you needed and did the best you could. I remember one man who bathed all the kids while his wife gave birth. Then after the delivery he brought her a cup of tea and a jam tart . . . he was exceptional! Mostly it was up to the women neighbours to help. . . .

(Midwife Mrs Shaw, working in the early 1900s, quoted in *Ordinary Lives*)

C For the 80% of women whose pregnancy is normal, the experience of childbirth could be a much more natural one. Obstetrics has never been very much interested in normal childbirth – which has always been left to the midwives – but has now concentrated on the pathological. The result is that by degrees normal childbirth in hospital has become pathologised. (Report by Louise and Oliver Gillie, *Sunday Times*, 24 October 1974)

D In ideal conditions I guess every woman should have a choice of home or hospital but I tend to agree . . . that primary importance should be put on changing, improving and extending the facilities and attitudes in hospitals under the National Health. I had to insist on having a full eight-days stay in the hospital after my second baby was born. I was determined to take advantage of being in the hospital to rest, get a few nights' full sleep and not worry or feel guilty about *anything* at home . . . With the exception of a few communes and women's houses, the home birth advocates, without actually saying so, rest their case on a 'happy family' base. (Sue O'Sullivan, letter to *Spare Rib*, August 1975)

Questions

1 Why were the untrained midwives referred to in A looked on with suspicion? Why did women consult them?
2 What are the advantages and disadvantages of having a baby at home, compared with going into hospital?

CHAPTER 9

Women and Health Today

Baroness Mary Warnock (b. 1924)

Mary Warnock's contribution to health has been largely in the field of medical ethics. Lady Warnock was educated at Oxford and in 1949 married a fellow philosopher, Geoffrey Warnock. She and her husband both obtained fellowships at Oxford, and Lady Warnock became the first married Fellow of St Hugh's College. The couple had five children, which meant that a good deal of domestic help was necessary. In an interview with Andrew Duncan, Lady Warnock said: 'I'm proud I didn't have to take time off'. (*Sunday Times*, May 1986). In 1966 she became headteacher of Oxford High School and since 1985 she has been Mistress of Girton College, Cambridge. Her husband is Principal of Hertford College, Oxford. The couple, however, have a home in Wiltshire, where they can be together at the weekends.

Lady Warnock feels that it is only by chance that she has been appointed to government committees:

> Once you are recognized, you are used as a specimen over and over again . . . I was put on a government list by Peter Shore, simply by chance because I knew his wife, and now I keep being pulled out. (*Sunday Times* interview, May 1986)

In the non-academic world, she has been a member of the IBA and, in the early 1970s, she chaired a government inquiry into special education for handicapped children. In 1981 she was on the Royal Commission on Environmental Polution and she has frequently spoken on health matters in the House of Lords.

I notice with despair and irritation in the Lords that, apart

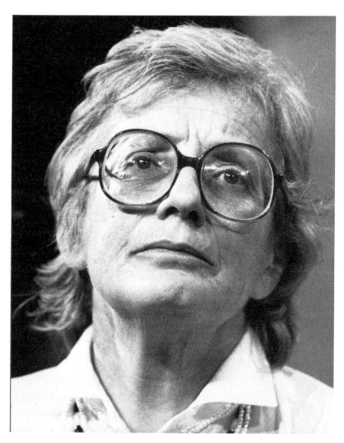

36 *Baroness Warnock, Chairperson of the Warnock Committee of Inquiry into Human Fertilization (1979-84).*

from Lady Young, women are not supposed to know about foreign policy or legal matters. It's always the caring subjects – children, education and health. (*Sunday Times* interview, May 1986)

It is as Chairman of the Warnock Committee of

Inquiry into Human Fertilization between 1979 and 1984 that Mary Warnock is best known.

> Mary Warnock's qualifications to preside over such a moral and legal minefield were a combination of academic distinction, long experience in teaching and public service, plus a ruthless common sense. (Suzanne Lowry, *Sunday Times*, June 1984)

Advances in science had created moral and social problems in medicine, particularly in areas dealing with abortion, test-tube babies and experimentation with human embryos. The committee consisted of 16 lay-people, doctors, scientists and theologians.

The committee's report recommended that a statutory authority should be set up to monitor test-tube baby research and other treatments for infertility and to control research on human embryos. Research on human embryos should be limited to 14 days after fertilization and beyond that should be a criminal offence.

> It seems *grotesque* that animal experimentation should be regulated by law, and that there should be no such law for human experimentation. (Lady Warnock, quoted in the *Sunday Times*, June 1984)

The commitee also suggested that legal changes should be introduced to make children born by artificial insemination or embryo donation legitimate. In certain circumstances, surrogate motherhood should be banned. Donors should remain anonymous and legislation introduced to remove any possible claim to parental rights. The committee differed on some points; for example the Catholic view was that no research at all should be allowed on embryos.

Questions

1 How did Mary Warnock become involved in the question of medical ethics?
2 Why are regulations necessary to control scientific intervention in pregnancy?

Equality in Health

It is now a century and a half since the first women doctors qualified. Today, women predominate in the total workforce of health-related professions, but few reach the top level of management. Women also make use of the National Health Service more often than men. A further problem for women is that medical technology is developing at a rapid rate, creating ethical problems, many of which are connected with bearing children.

Although nearly half the entrants to medical school today are women, only two per cent become surgeons. Until recently the female intake was restricted on the grounds that there was always a 'wastage' element due to marriage and children. Dr Elizabeth Shore remembers when she was training in the 1940s:

> There were only five women out of sixty students in my year so you got a disproportionate amount of attention, and had to know things and be on your toes. I remember one consultant asking me, 'Is your husband dead?' These men had never *seen* women medical students before. (Quoted in *The Compleat Woman*)

When the Equal Opportunities Bill was passed in 1975, and Elizabeth Shore was working at the Department of Health and Social Security (DHSS), she noticed that most London hospitals and Oxbridge still worked a quota system for women, keeping the intake down to about 20 per cent a year. After she had her fourth child she herself had found it easier to work in a clinic because the hours were better. When the children became older, she went to the DHSS and rose to the rank of Deputy Secretary – a higher grade than any other woman with children had reached in the Civil Service at that time.

Even today, most women do not stay the course to become surgeons as they will have to be hospital-based and working anti-social hours until they are well over 30, a time of life when they often have domestic commitments or are thinking of starting a family. In

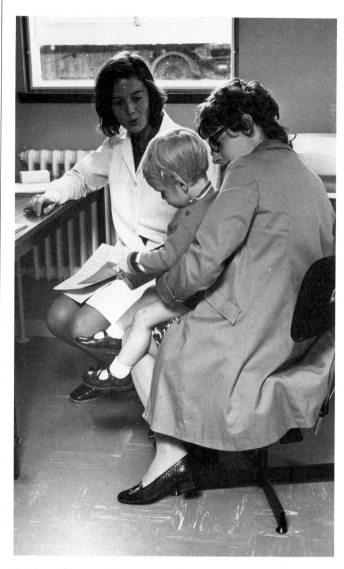

37 A mother consults a woman doctor at a health clinic, 1971. Many women doctors find it convenient to work part-time in such clinics.

1987 Wendy Savage described how there were no female professors of obstetrics or gynaecology, 'although this is a specialty dealing exclusively with women' (*Women in Medicine*, from *Medicine in Contemporary Society*, edited by Peter Byrne). According to tables collated in 1985, only 0.6 per cent of consultants in general surgery were women, 4.3 per cent in general medicine, 11.5 per cent in geriatric medicine, 18.6 per cent paediatrics, 18.8 per cent in anaesthetics and 37 per cent in child psychiatry. Although 20.3 per cent of senior registrars were women, only 11.6 per cent went on to become consultants.

On the other hand, 20 per cent of doctors in general practice and psychiatry are women, and community medicine is also popular with them. Almost all female doctors continue to practise medicine, although many married women are part-timers for at least a short period in their careers, often working as child health doctors or in Family Planning and Well-Woman clinics. A British Medical Association (BMA) working party report in May 1989 recommended that part-time training posts should be established at every level and that the quality of the training should be monitored. It was also suggested that employers should provide better child-care facilities. In dentistry, females are still in the minority, although abroad this is not the case; in Eastern Europe, in particular, almost 80 per cent of dentists are women. On the other hand, dental hygienists and surgery assistants are more often female.

Nursing has remained a predominately female profession. Although between 1974 and 1984 nurses had more chance of getting top jobs in management, since the Health Service changes in 1984 the opportunities have decreased and poor pay is a constant source of grievance. Women predominate in the professions allied to medicine – physiotherapy, occupational and speech therapy, radiography, dietetics – but are poorly paid.

In hospitals, two-thirds of the ancillary staff (domestic staff, laundry and catering workers) are women, as are most of the clerical staff. In the community, home nurses, health visitors and home helps are almost always female, as are most of hospital and home based social workers – although men generally have the top jobs. The number of women employed in pharmacy is rising, and the Pharmaceutical Society has a woman president, Mrs Margaret Rawlings. Sixty per cent of the 1989 intake to the profession was female, a trend which reflects the ease with which the work can be fitted in with domestic commitments.

Some very dedicated women have managed to rise to the top of the medical profession. Although women have been under-represented in the professional bodies – the Royal Colleges, the General Medical Council (GMC) and the British Medical Association (BMA) – the situation is improving gradually.

Dr Margaret Turner-Warwick was elected in March 1989 as the first woman president of the Royal College of Physicians. Dr Beulah Bewley, epidemiologist and

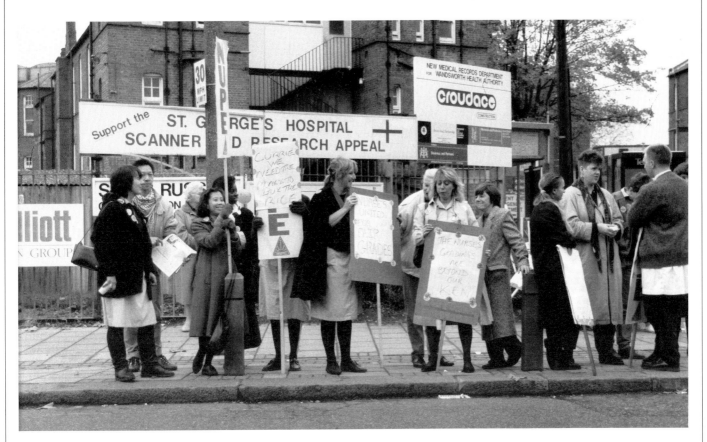

38 *Nurses strike for more pay at St George's Hospital, London, 1988.*

specialist in community medicine, now president of the Medical Women's Federation, was made a member of the GMC after writing a paper asking about the misuse of woman power in hospitals and the lack of representation for women on professional bodies.

The eminent obstetrician and gynaecologist Dame Josephine Barnes was Vice President of the Royal College of Obstetricians and Gynaecologists from 1977 to 1978 and the first woman President of the BMA (1979-80). Dame Rosemary Rue was the President elect for 1989-90. There has only been one female president of the British Dental Association, Lilian Lindsay.

Some women have been influential in the management of the Health Service as specialists in community medicine, at the Department of Health (DOH) or at regional and district levels. The running of the National Health Service (NHS) locally is under the control of Regional and District Health Authorities which represent professional and local interests. The members come from all walks of life and there is a large percentage of women.

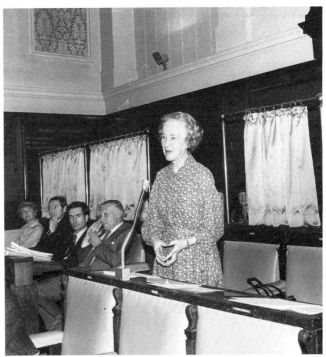

39 *Dame Josephine Barnes at the 1981 BMA Council Meeting. Dame Josephine was the first woman President of the Association (1979-80).*

Community physician Dame Rosemary Rue, who was made President of the Faculty of Community Medicine in 1986, was Regional Medical Officer and then Regional General Manager of the Oxford Health Authority until her retirement in 1988. Dame Alison Munro was Chairman of the Merton, Sutton and Wandsworth Area Health Authority between 1964 and 1974, Governor of the Charing Cross Group of Hospitals from 1973 to 1981 and Chairman of the Chichester Health Authority between 1982 and 1988. Julia Cumberlege became Chairman of the Brighton Health Authority in 1981 and Chairman of the South West Thames Regional Health Authority in 1989. She also chaired a review of Community Nursing in 1985 and has worked in an Advisory Group on AIDs. Dr Elizabeth Shaw, after a top appointment in the DHSS (now DOH), is now Dean of the North West Thames region of the British Postgraduate Medical Federation of the University of London.

One of the most important steps concerning women's health was the foundation of the Women's National Cancer Control Campaign by MP Mrs Joyce Butler in 1964, with Dame Josephine Barnes as President. The Campaign believes in alerting women to the dangers of cancer through health education and screening, provides mobile clinics for cervical screening and is now raising money for mobile mammography units.

> All these intiatives are working towards the same end. Our attempts to encourage women to have as much control over their own health as they possibly can. (Sara McKenzie, Director Women's National Cancer Control Campaign.)

During the first half of the nineteenth century, the pioneers of women's liberation were trying to prove that women could do the same jobs as men and were not on average significantly different in their physical capabilities. In contrast, the last 25 years have seen the growth of various voluntary bodies and self-help groups run by women, specifically concerned with female health problems. An example is the Pre-menstrual Tension Advisory Service founded by Maryon Stewart. The danger of making women into a special case is that society might again decide that they need protection from certain kinds of work which they are perfectly capable of performing.

The present trend in health for both sexes is towards prevention and self-help. We certainly now know much more about the workings of our bodies than our

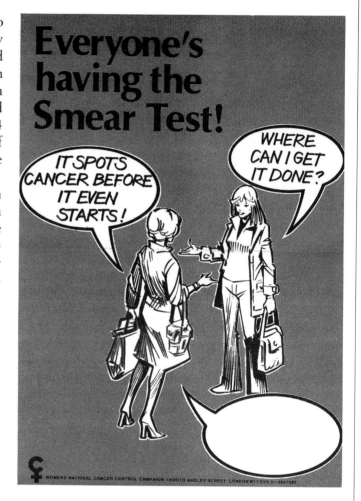

40 *Publicity from the Women's National Cancer Control Campaign.*

grandparents did and are more health conscious. There has also been a trend during the 1980s towards alternative and holistic medicine (which looks at the whole person rather than the local disease process). This may well be a reaction against the very technological nature of conventional medicine today. These skills are not state-registered and so cannot be obtained through the NHS. They include acupuncture, homeopathic medicine (whose practitioners try to attack a disease by stimulating the body's natural defences) and osteopathy (which deals with joint and muscle problems). A large percentage of the followers of alternative medicine are women. *Spare Rib* attributes this to the way women have been treated by male doctors in the past, particularly in gynaecological matters.

Most women still seem to prefer to consult other women about specifically female medical problems, and some of their needs are catered for by female GPs and the Well-Woman clinics. Dame Josephine Barnes, who was a consultant at the all-female Elizabeth Garrett Anderson Hospital in London for a great many years, believes:

> The principle of women-only hospitals is a good thing. We get a lot of women who dislike being treated by a man, women of all ages. We take great pains to see they are sympathetically received, told what is wrong and generally treated like human beings. (Quoted in the *Guardian*, 11 August 1978)

After a long campaign to stop its closure, the Elizabeth Garrett Anderson Hospital merged with the Hospital for Women, Soho in 1989, changing its policy of employing only women doctors. Now men are also on the staff, but patients are free to choose the doctor they prefer.

Medical technology, new diseases and different methods of dealing with them have made health matters more complex today than they were fifty years ago. Women also take part in research projects, like Dr Ros Angel, whose field is embryo research. It has been proved statistically that if an open access medical service is offered specifically to women, a greater number of female problems come to light. The same applies to the population as a whole. This free medical treatment and open access, which have been provided by the National Health Service for over 40 years, should not be relinquished without very good reason.

Evidence

A Some of the young male medical students are realising it's good to be a partner in the sharing and caring of children and instead of struggling up the hierarchy they opt for general practice. It's easier for women now, I think, to get to a consultancy first, say by age thirty-two, and then think about babies – but that has its problems . . . The clash between family and duty has to be resolved, by careful forward planning and by arranging adequate domestic cover. (Dr Beulah Bewley, senior lecturer and consultant epidemiologist, interview by Valerie Grove in *The Compleat Woman*)

B More than 60% of women (and a few men) know the miseries of recurrent cystitis. Four out of five women suffer from it at some time in their lives. Yet 80% of attacks are unwittingly self-caused and can be self-helped. Doctors have fobbed women off with antibiotics and operations without making them well. Now we have a new generation of doctors who are willing to let me prove what they all know in their hearts to be true . . . Here am I, a person with no medical training, let loose among them to conduct trials which do not deal in drugs, only commonsense and scrupulous hygiene. What is more, they see the patients doing half the work and obviously enjoying themselves . . . There is a real feeling among the women that they are participating in their own health care. There is no reason why the medical profession should not dispense with some of its formality. (Angela Kilmartin, pioneer in the treatment of cystitis, now conducting research at University College London's Institute of Urology; interviewed in the *Sunday Times*, 6 November 1988)

C Three years ago Mary Beth Whitehead rented her womb to Bill and Betsy Sterns for roughly 60 cents an hour. As a surrogate mother, she carried Sara, later to become known as Baby M, and when the child was born what she found herself wanting more than anything else was the right to keep the child. (Report in the *Guardian*, 13 February 1990. After appeal, the Sterns kept the baby and the natural mother was given parental and visiting rights. Surrogacy was then banned in New Jersey, USA.)

Questions

1 Why do woman doctors find it difficult to qualify as consultants? Are there similar problems in any other professions?

2 With reference to B, explain why many women are dissatisfied with conventional medicine. Do you think health care should be left to doctors and nurses?

3 Explain the moral and legal problem expressed in C. Why do you think Mary Beth Whitehead wanted to keep the baby?

Timeline

1812	A woman masquerading as James Barry qualifies as a doctor.
1849	Elizabeth Blackwell qualifies as a doctor in America.
1851	Amelia Bloomer's reformed dress for women arrives in Britain.
1854-6	Crimean War: Female nurses are authorized to work in army hospitals.
1860	Nightingale School for training nurses opens in London.
1865	Elizabeth Garrett qualifies as a doctor (Society of Apothecaries exam).
1869	First women students admitted by the Edinburgh Medical School.
1902	The Midwives Act is passed.
1903	Bedford Physical Training College for Women opens in London.
1914-18	First World War widens women's civil & military employment prospects.
1916	*Married Love* by Marie Stopes is published.
1919	Nurses Registration Act.
1921	Marie Stopes opens the first Birth Control clinic in London.
1928	First women take part in the Olympic Games.
1930	Women's League of Health and Beauty founded.
1931	National Birth Control Association formed.
1939	Family Planning Association formed.
1939-45	Second World War: First atomic bombs dropped in 1945.
1948	National Health Service Act.
1955	Women's National Cancer Control Campaign formed by Joyce Butler.
1957	British hydrogen bomb tested. First Aldermaston March.
1962	Environmentalist Rachel Carson publishes *Silent Spring*.
1963	Betty Frieden writes *The Feminine Mystique*.
1964	Brook Advisory Centres opens to advise unmarried women on contraception.
1967	Abortion Act enables termination of pregnancy on health grounds, with medical consent.
1971	First Chiswick Women's Aid Centre opens for battered wives.
1975	Equal Opportunities Bill passed.
1976	Women's Therapy Centre opens in London.
1979	Dame Josephine Barnes becomes the first Woman President of the British Medical Association.
1984	Women are allowed to run the Olympic marathon for the first time.
1985	Wendy Savage is suspended from the London Hospital for her obstetric beliefs.
1986	The Suzy Lamplugh Trust is founded to protect women at work.
1987	Start of the Women's Environmental Network.
1989	Dr Margaret Turner-Warwick is elected first woman president of the Royal College of Physicians.
1990	Baroness Warnock's Report on Human Fertilization.

Books for further reading

Carol Adam, *Ordinary Lives*, Virago, 1982

Rachel Carson, *The Silent Spring*, Hamish Hamilton 1963

Rachel Carson, *The Sea Around Us*, Staples Press, 1951

Edmonde Charles-Roux, *Chanel*, Collins Harvill, 1989

Nigel Dudley, *This Poisoned Earth*, Judy Piatkus, 1987

John Elkington & Julia Hailes, *The Green Consumer Guide* , Victor Gollancz, 1988

Sheila Fletcher, *Women First*, The Athlone Press, 1984

Heather Flint, *Health & Welfare*, Batsford, 1983

Betty Friedan, *The Feminine Mystique*, Victor Gollancz, 1963

Charles N. Gattey, *The Bloomer Girls*, Macdonald, 1967

Barbara Griggs, *The Food Factor*, Viking, 1986

Valerie Grove, *The Compleat Woman*, The Hogarth Press, 1988

Ruth Hall, *Marie Stopes: A Biography*, Andre Deutsch, 1973

Ruth Hall (ed.), *Dear Dr Stopes*, Andre Deutsch, 1978

Michael Hiley, *Victorian Working Women*, Gordon Fraser Gallery, 1979

Liz Hodgkinson, *Addictions*, Thorsons Publishing Group, 1986

Pat Hodgson, *Working Lives: Nursing*, Batsford, 1986

Angela Holdsworth, *Out of the Doll's House*, BBC Books, 1988

Charles Kightly, *Country Voice*, Thames & Hudson, 1984

Sheila Kitzinger, *The Midwife Challenge*, Pandora, 1988

Joyce Leeson & Judith Gray, *Woman and Medicine*, Tavistock Publications, 1978

Diana Lamplugh, *Survive the 9-5*, Grapevine, 1988

Arthur Marwick, *Beauty in History*, Thames & Hudson, 1988

Kathleen E. McCrone, *Sport and the Physical Emancipation of English Women*, Routledge, 1988

Susie Orbach, *Hunger Strike*, Faber & Faber, 1987

Susie Orbach, *Fat Is a Feminist Issue*, Paddington Press, 1978

Marguerite Patten, *We'll Eat Again*, Hamlyn Publishing, 1985

Ann Oakley, *The Captured Womb*, Basil Blackwell, 1984

Erin Pizzey, *Scream Quietly or the Neighbours will Hear*, IF Books, 1974

Erin Pizzey, *Infernal Child*, Victor Gollancz, 1978

Jonathon Porritt & David Winner, *The Coming of the Greens*, Fontana, 1988

Philippa Pullar, *Consuming Passions*, Hamish Hamilton, 1970

Wendy Savage, *A Savage Enquiry*, Virago, 1986

Edward Shorter, *A History of Women's Bodies*, Allen Lane, 1983

Prunella Stack, *Zest for Life*, Peter Owen, 1988

Andrew Stephen, *The Suzy Lamplugh Story*, Faber & Faber, 1988

Mary Stott (ed.), *Women Talking*, Pandora Press, 1987

Sue O'Sullivan (ed.), *Women's Health: A Spare Rib Reader*, Pandora Press, 1987

Reay Tannahill, *Food in History*, Penguin, 1973

Cecil Woodham Smith, *Florence Nightingale*, Constable, 1950

C.J.S. Thompson, *The Quacks of Old London*, Brentano, 1928

Index